Birth of The

New

BY

SOPHIA LEAH

Birth of The New
is Sophia Leah's fourth journal.
Antidepressants:
explosions of a
frustrated mind, Sophia's World
Tour, and
NAKED NATURE are also
available.

Please Contact
SOPHIA LEAH via:

mysecretsophia@yahoo.com

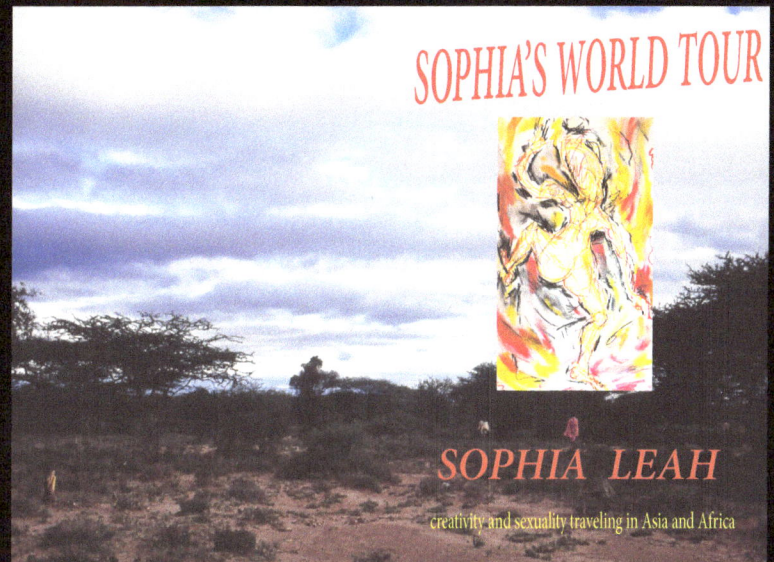

SOPHIA'S WORLD TOUR

SOPHIA LEAH

creativity and sexuality traveling in Asia and Africa

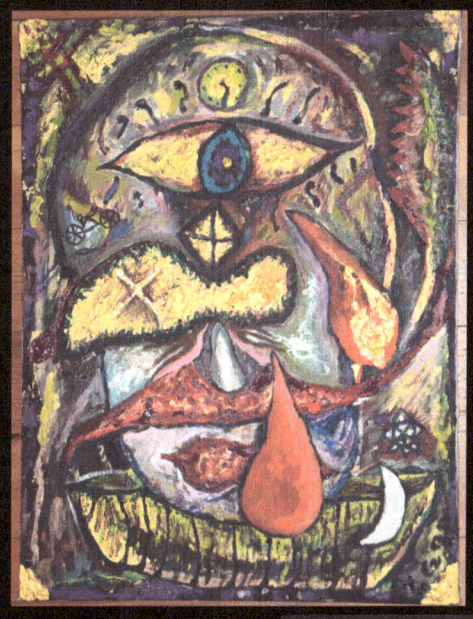

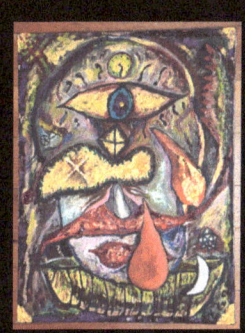

Antidepressants:

explosions from a frustrated mind

volume#1

Sophia Leah

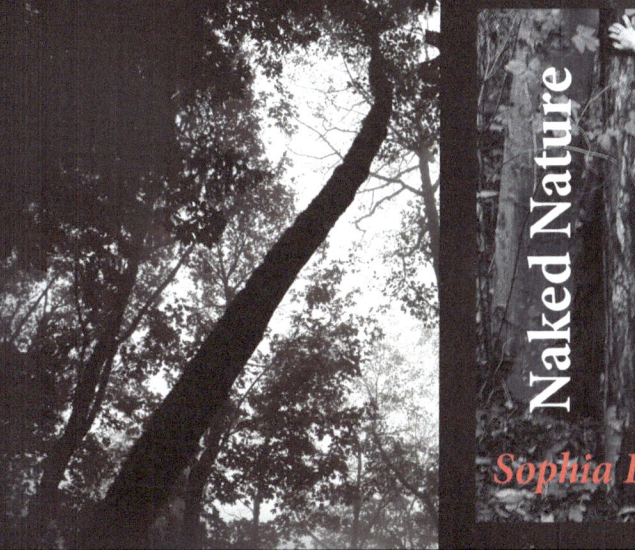

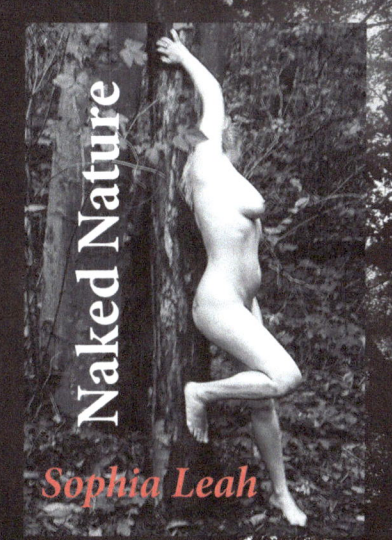

Naked Nature

Sophia Leah

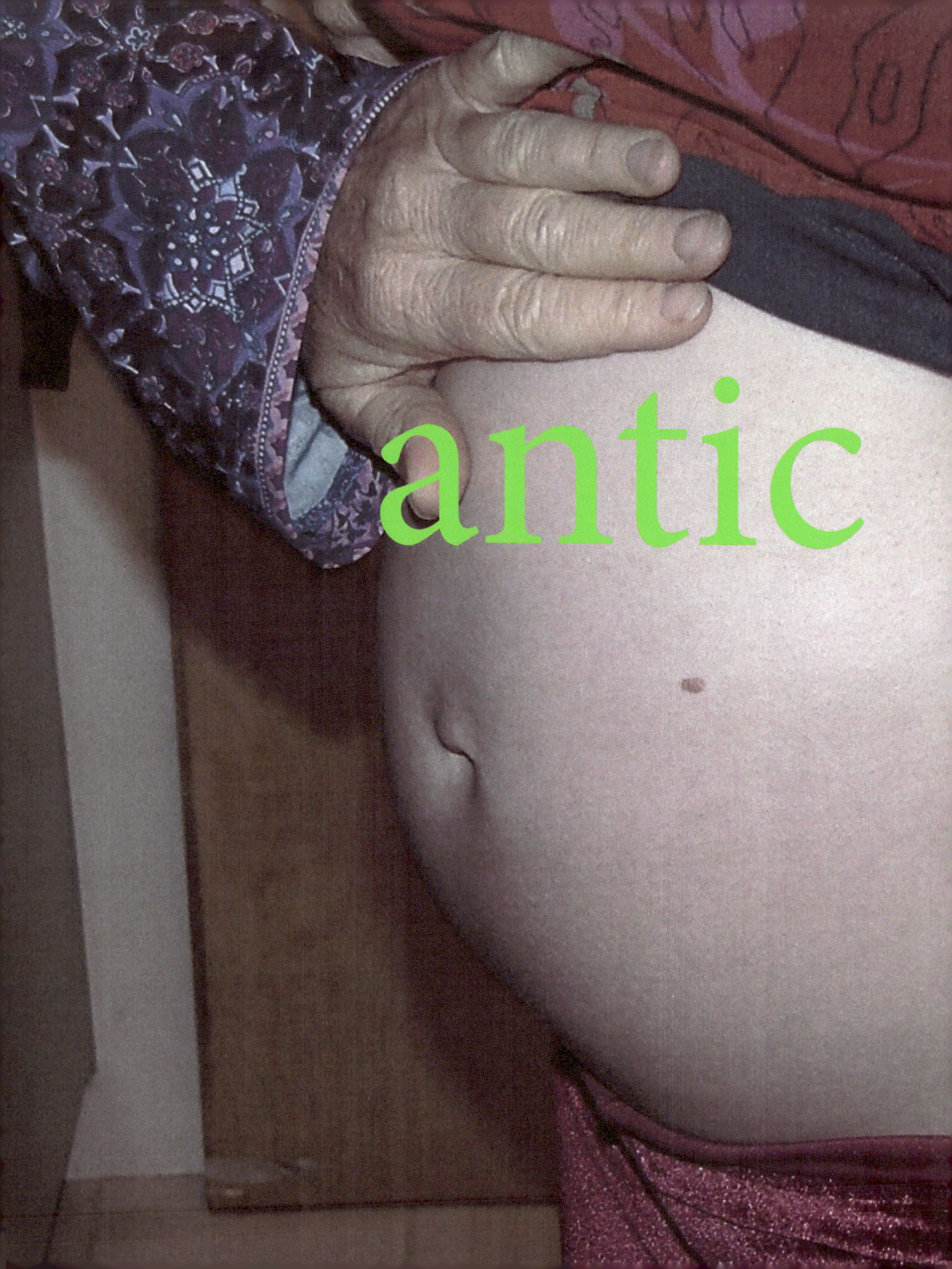

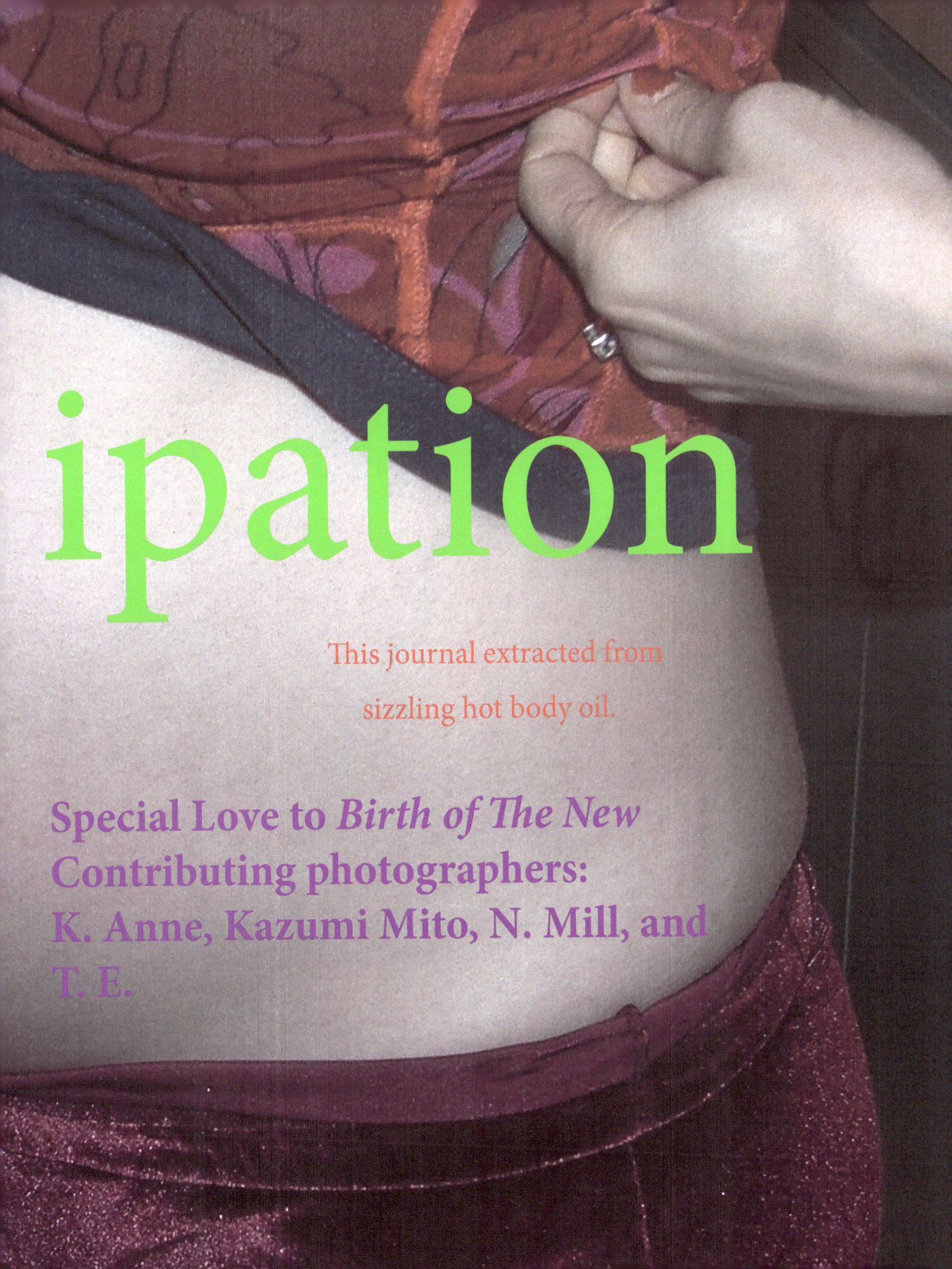

ipation

This journal extracted from
sizzling hot body oil.

Special Love to *Birth of The New*
Contributing photographers:
K. Anne, Kazumi Mito, N. Mill, and
T. E.

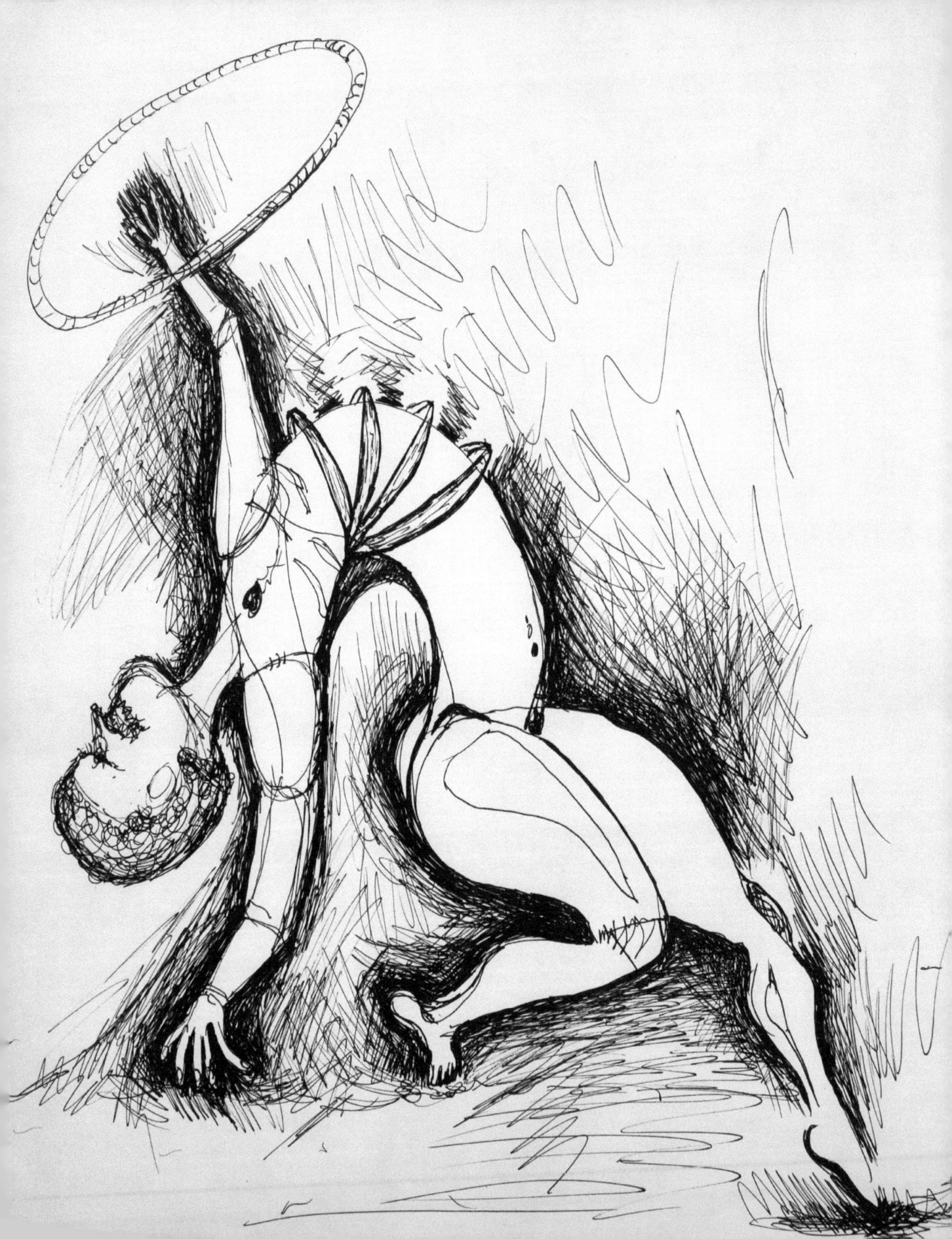

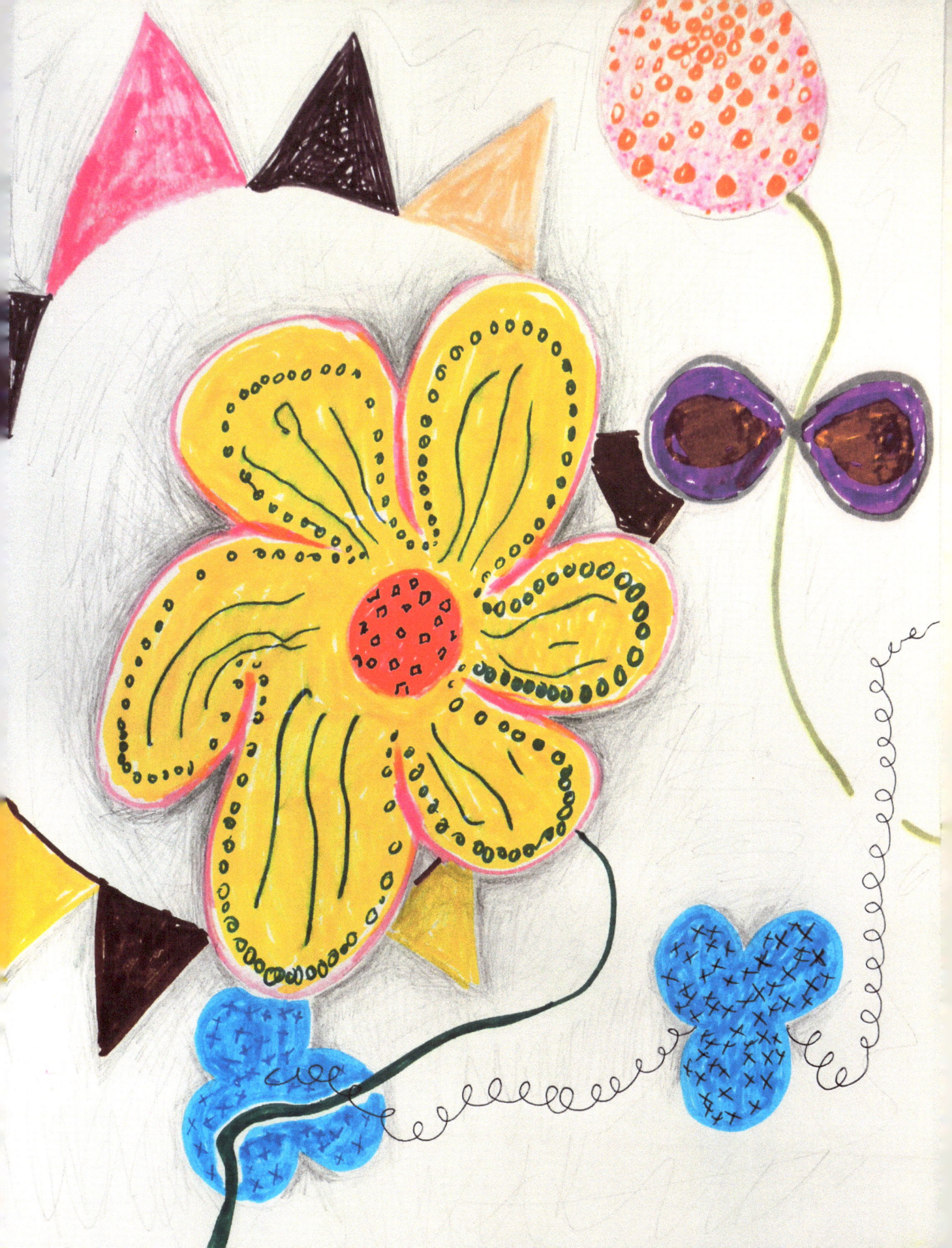

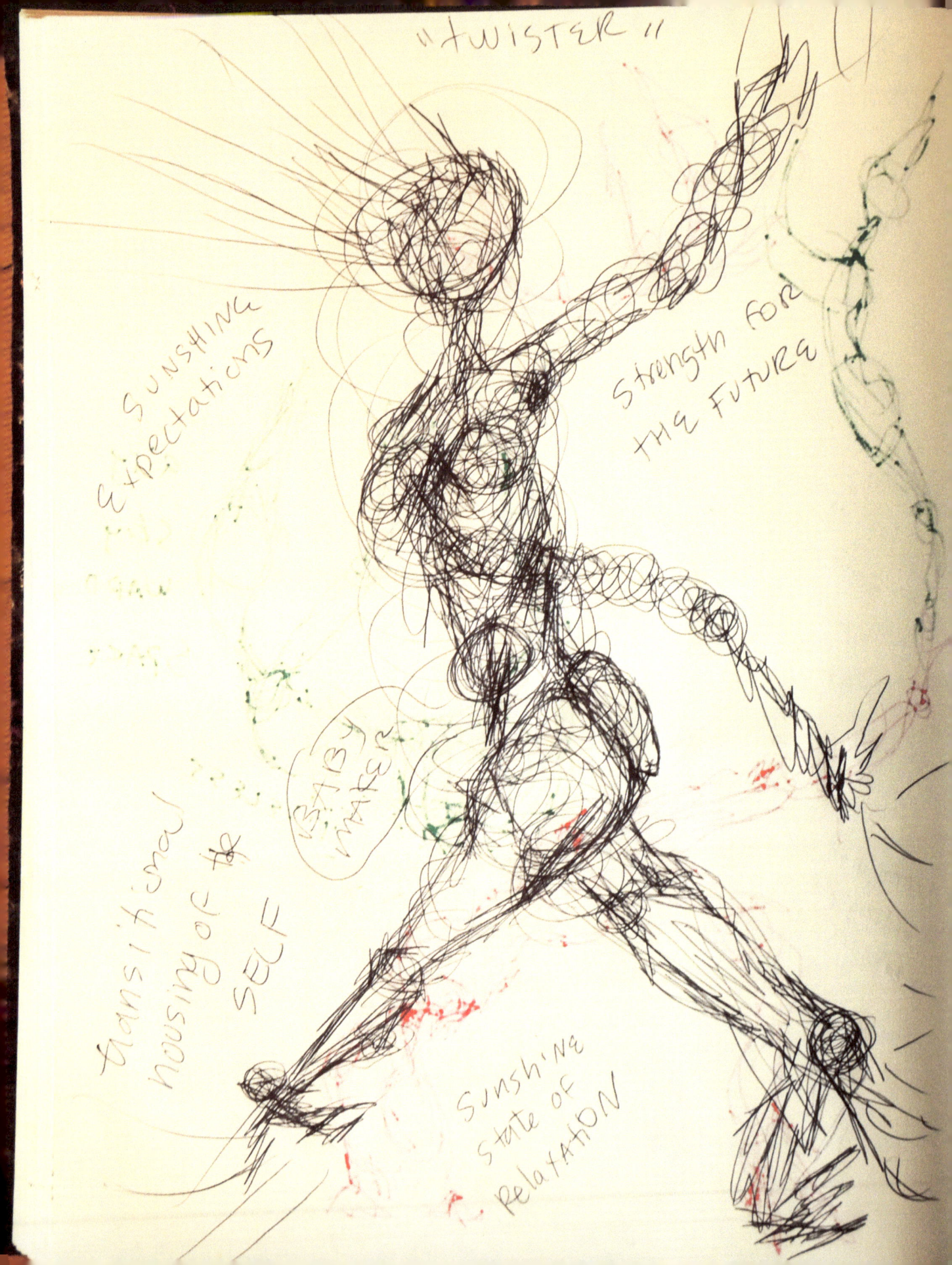

memories

WATER

CHARGE

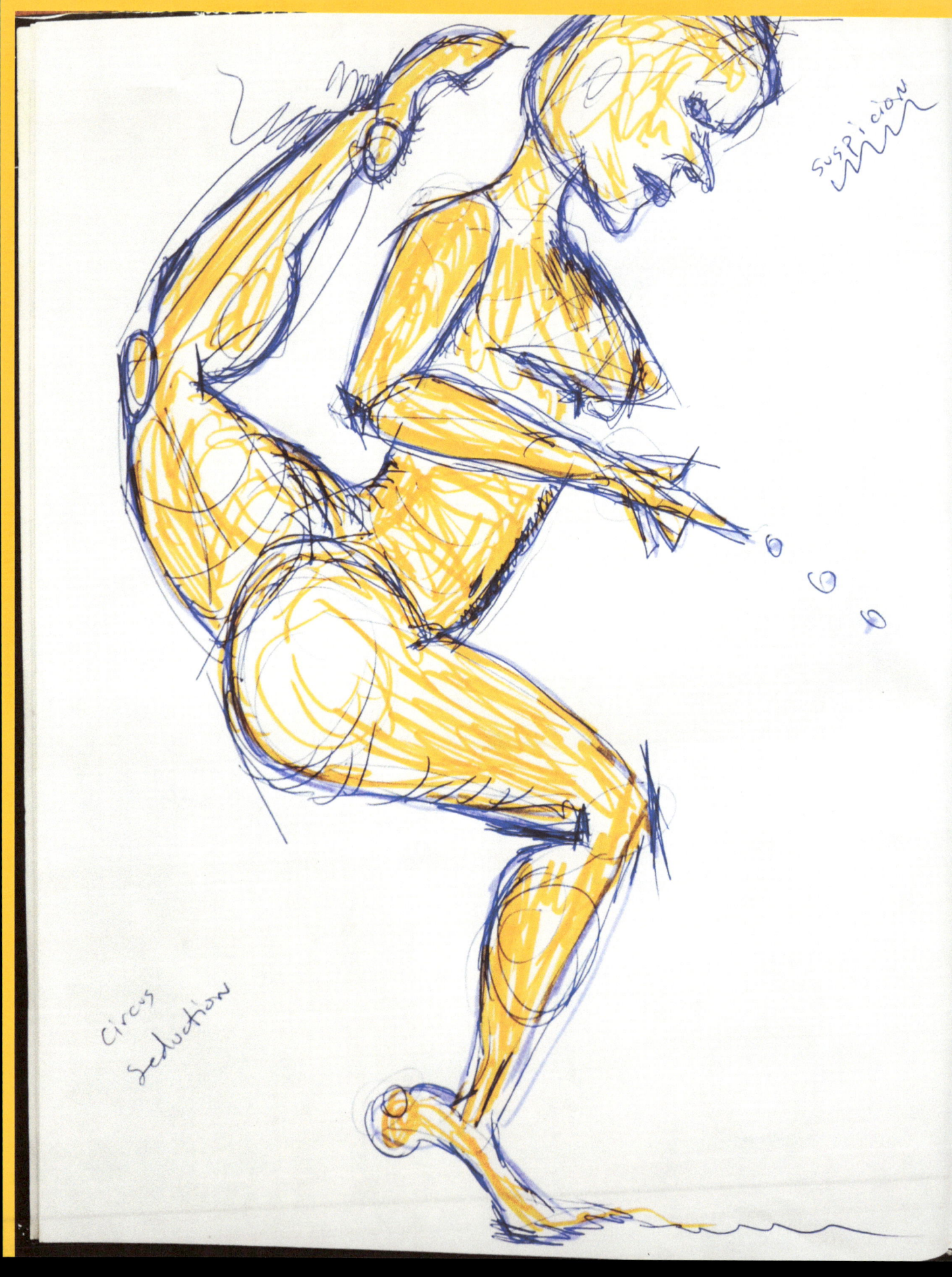

Suspicion

Circus
Seduction

Growth is something that happens suddenly or just flies like the wind. Birth is thought about fantasy but then what happens... A smell of something, a dream. Like 2 different worlds colliding... a birth a new IDEA always a change. BIRTH ~ cataclysmic OF COURSE! the Aftermath can be death or just survival of the fittest... or more love which is the HOPED for outcome.

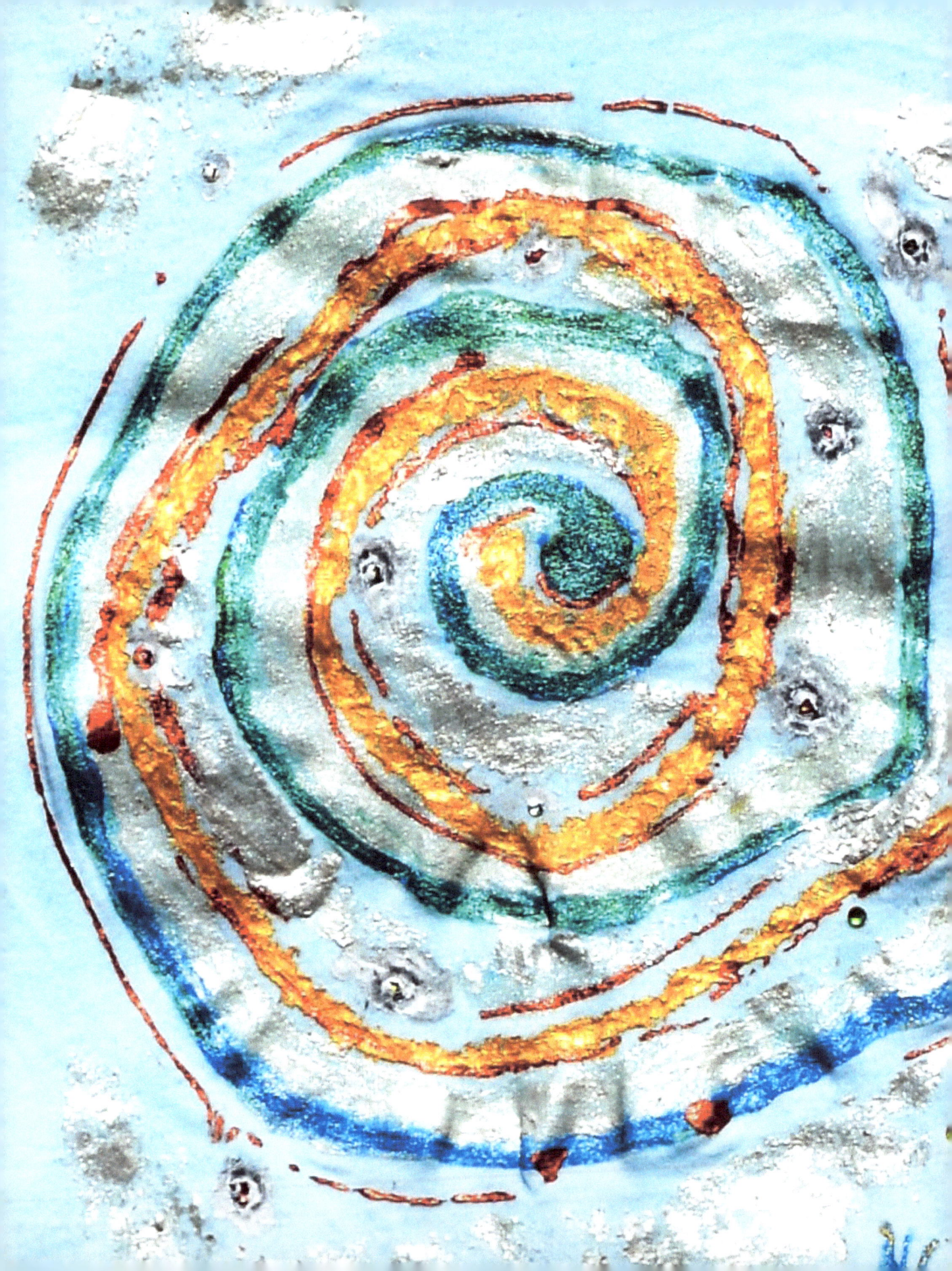

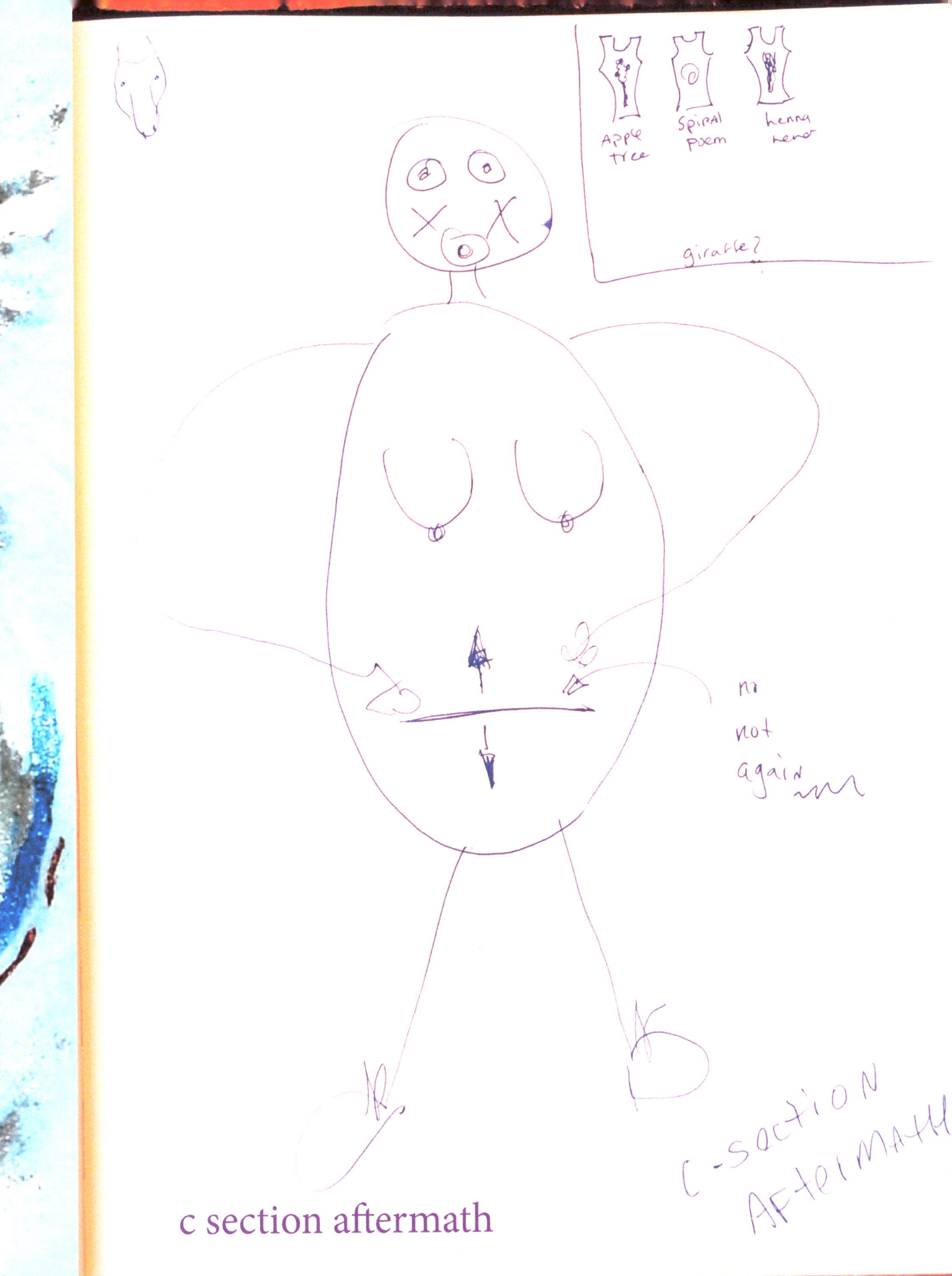

Apple tree   Spiral Poem   henna hend

giraffe?

no
not
again

c section aftermath

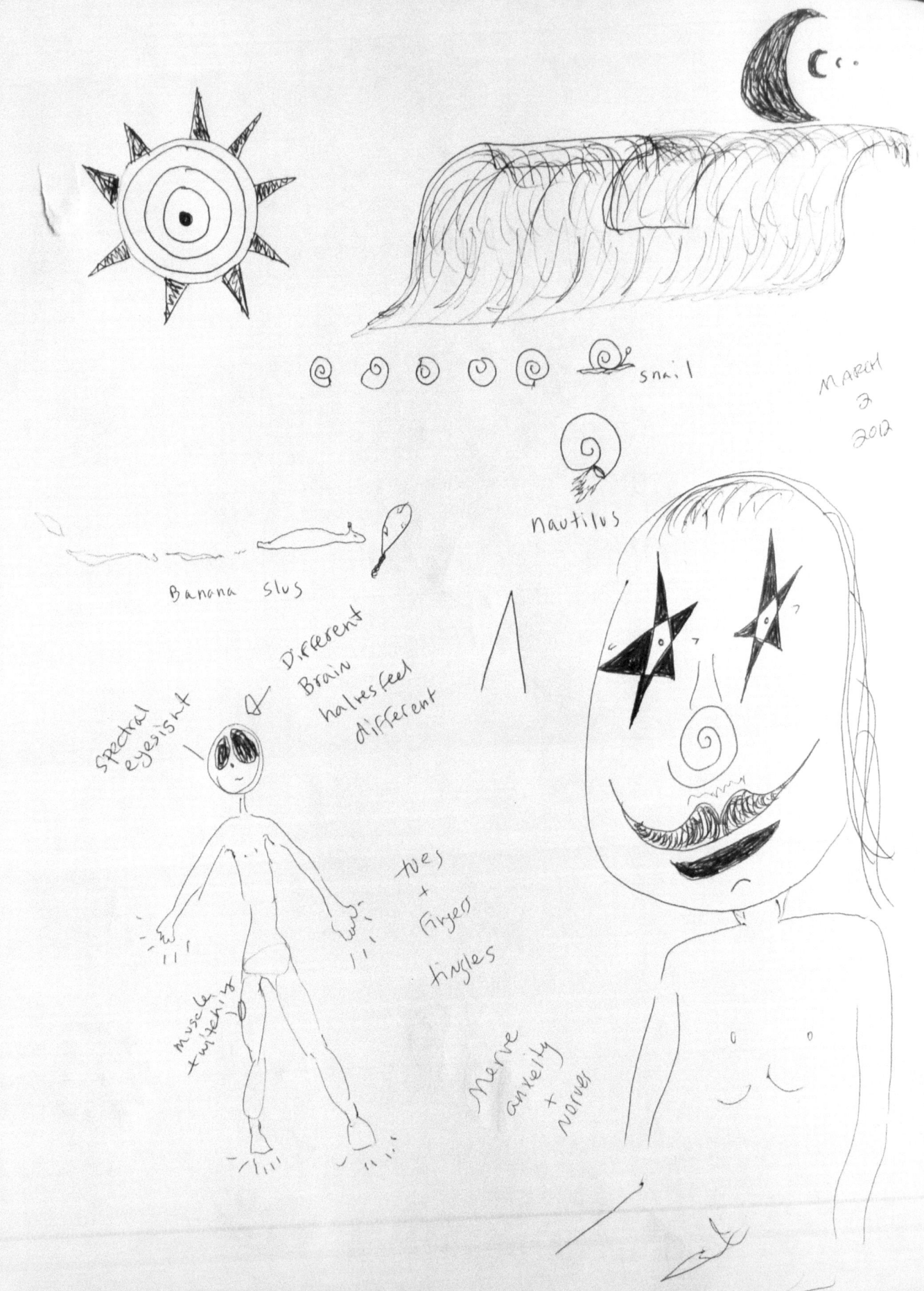

snail

MARCH
3
2012

nautilus

Banana slug

Different
Brain
halves feel
different

Spectral
eyesight

toes
+
fingers
tingles

muscle
twitching

Nerve
anxiety
+
nerves

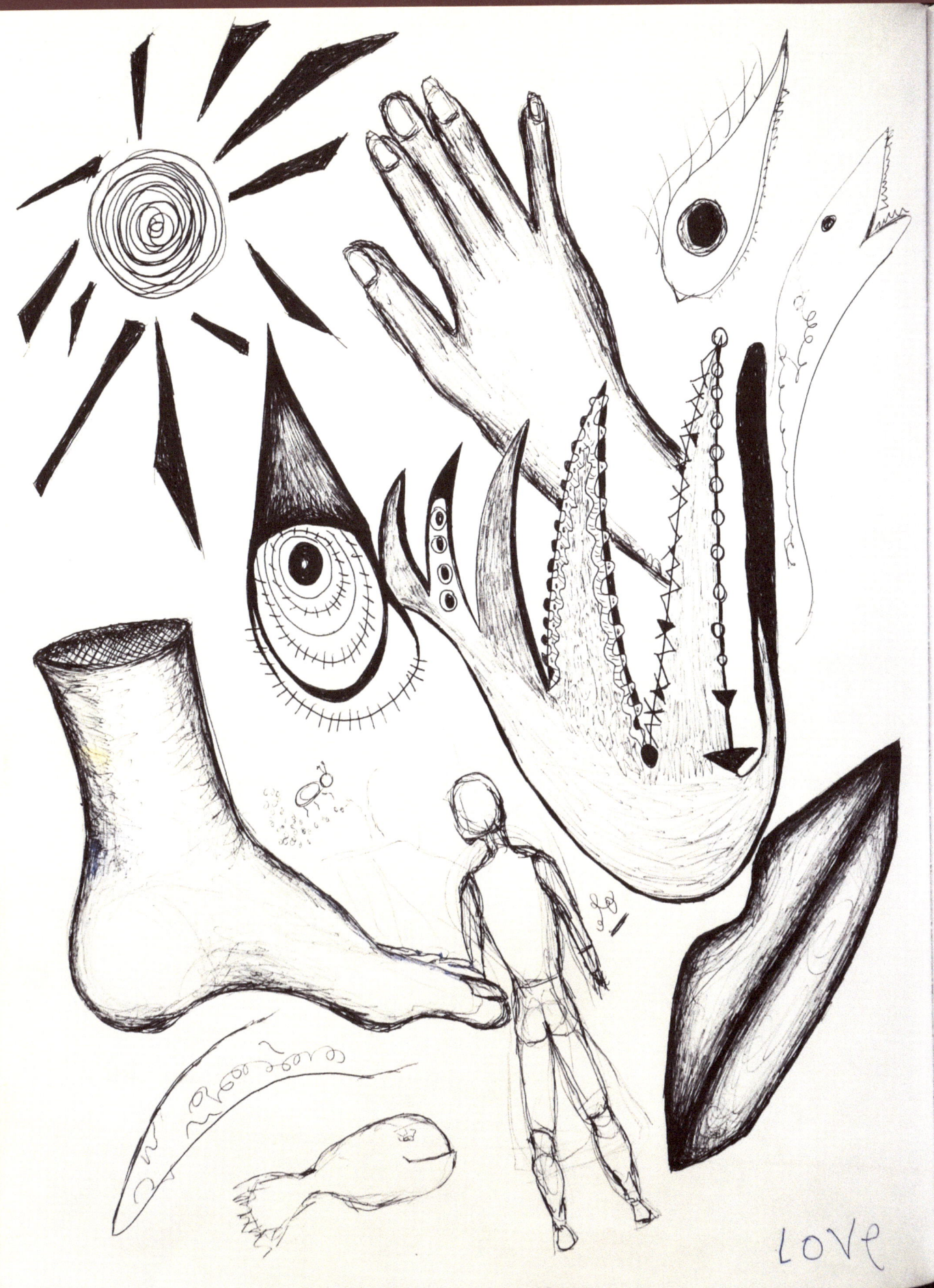

LOVe

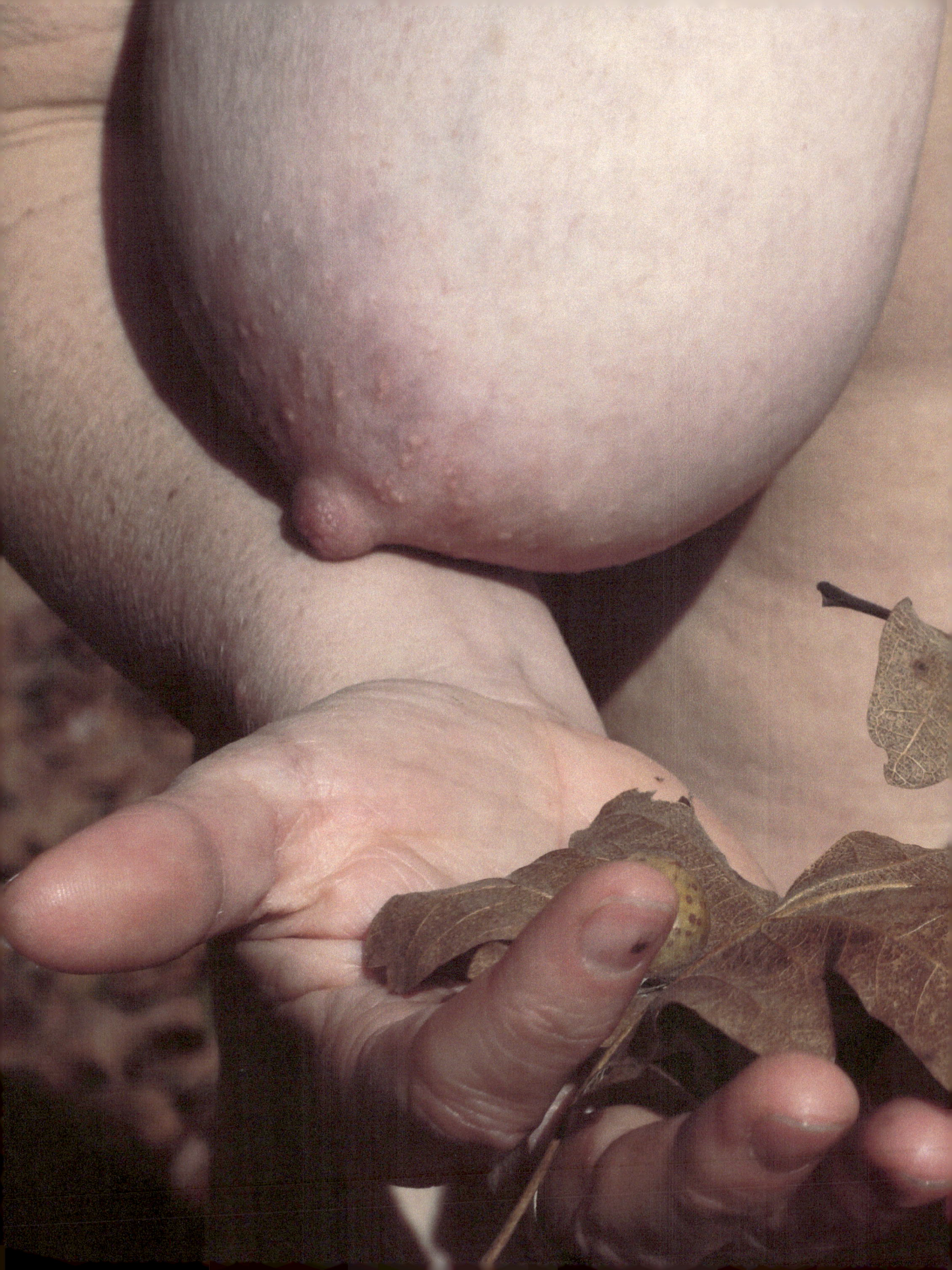

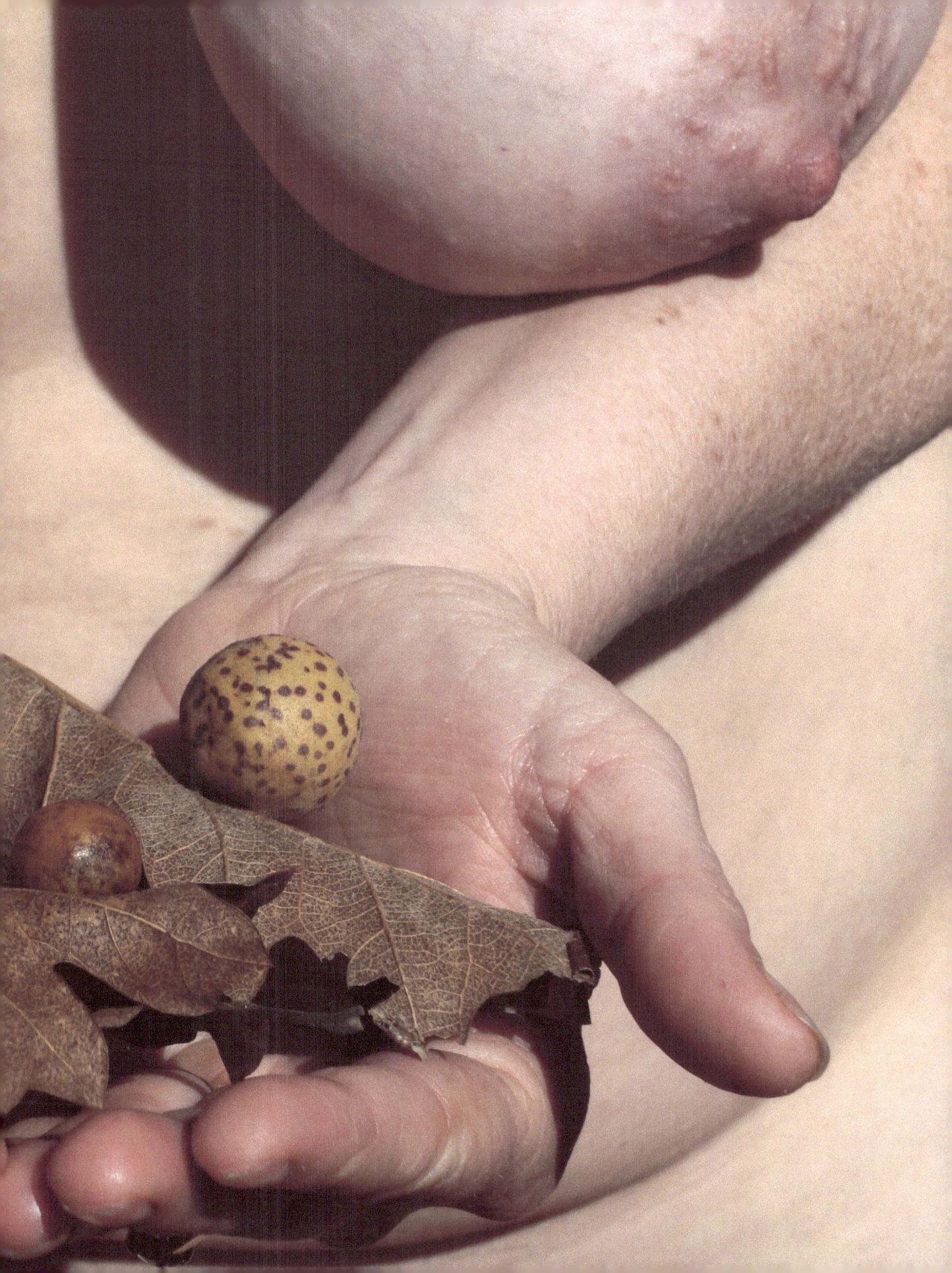

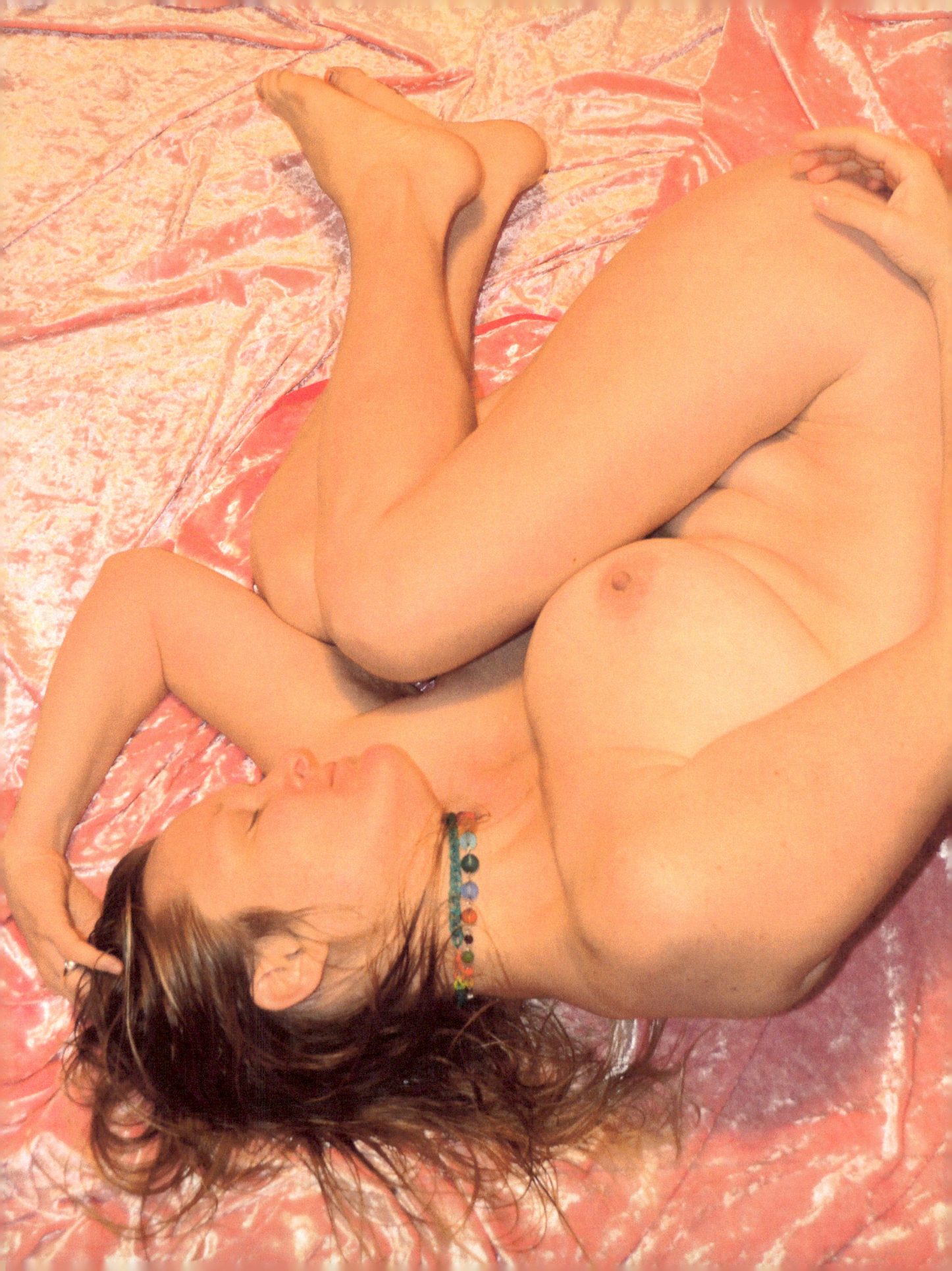

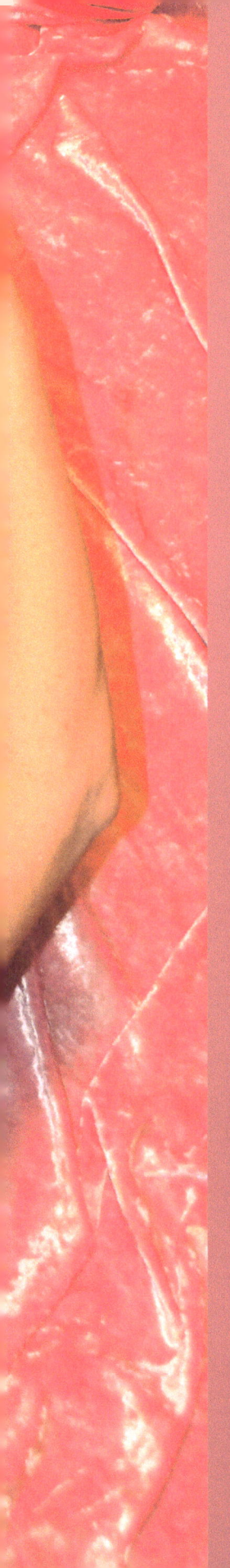

I am an egg of creation.

I create life.

COnstantly reworking

regrouping

Fresh out of the womb

BIRTH succumbs to death

Repeat

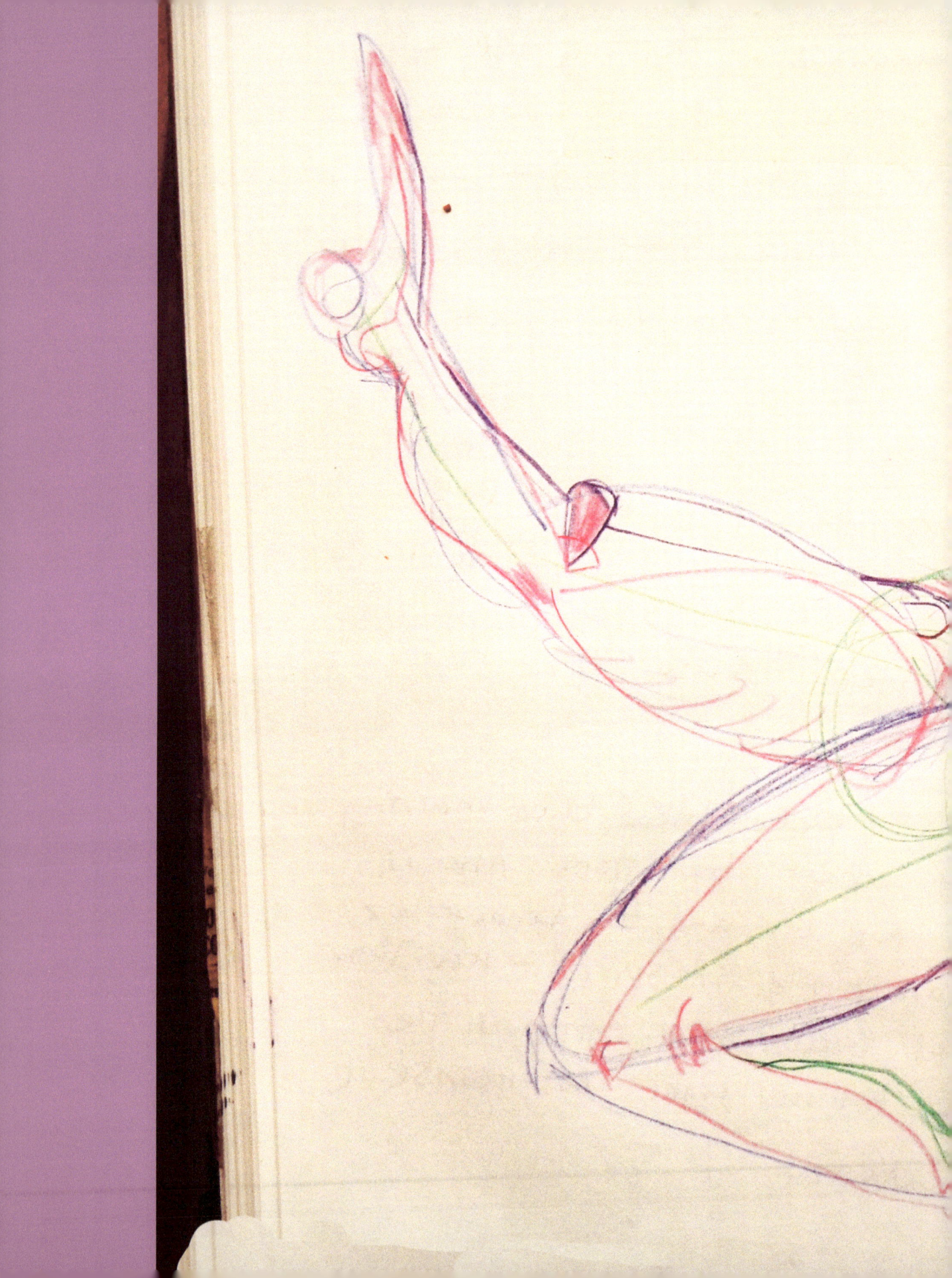

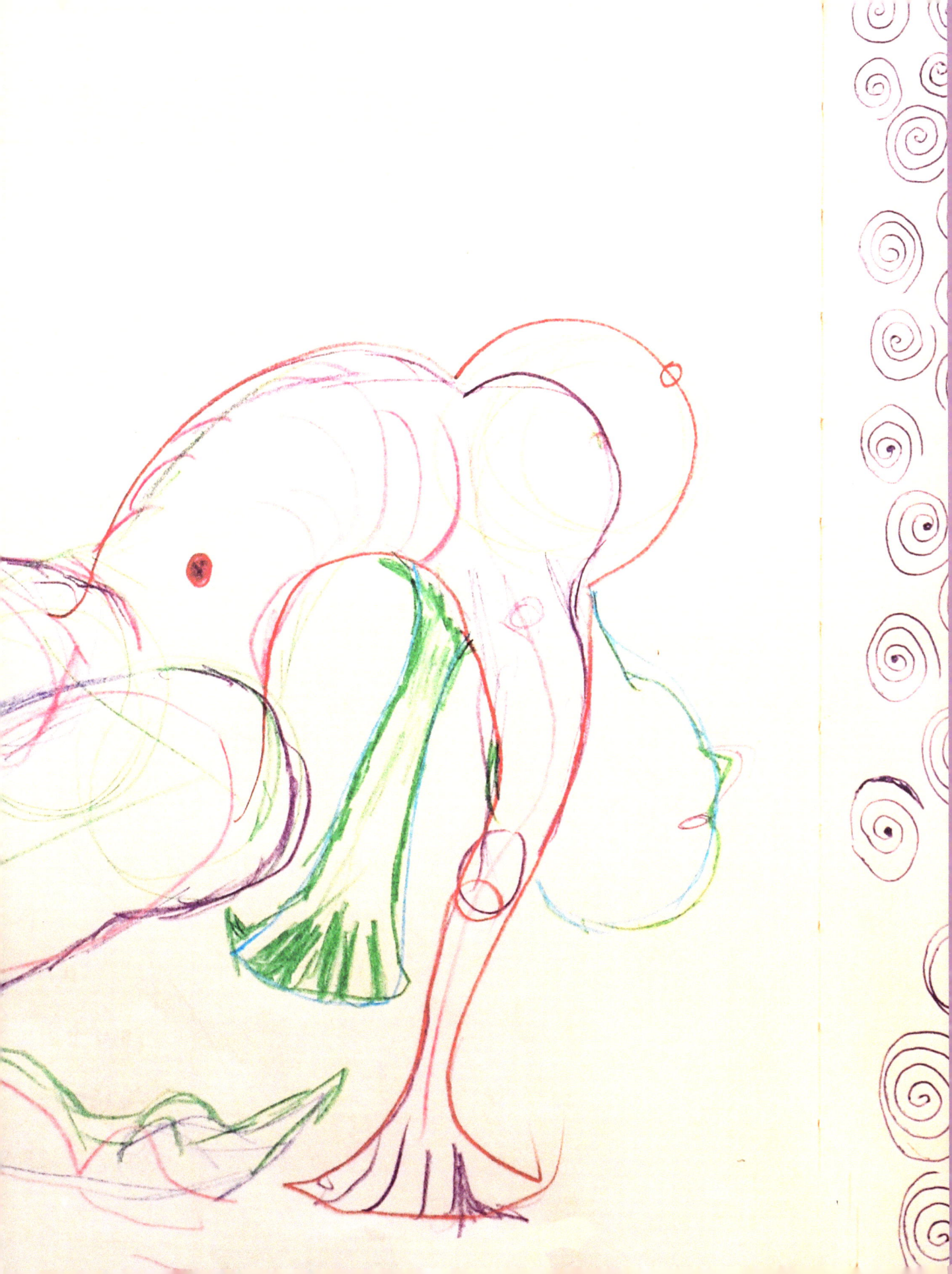

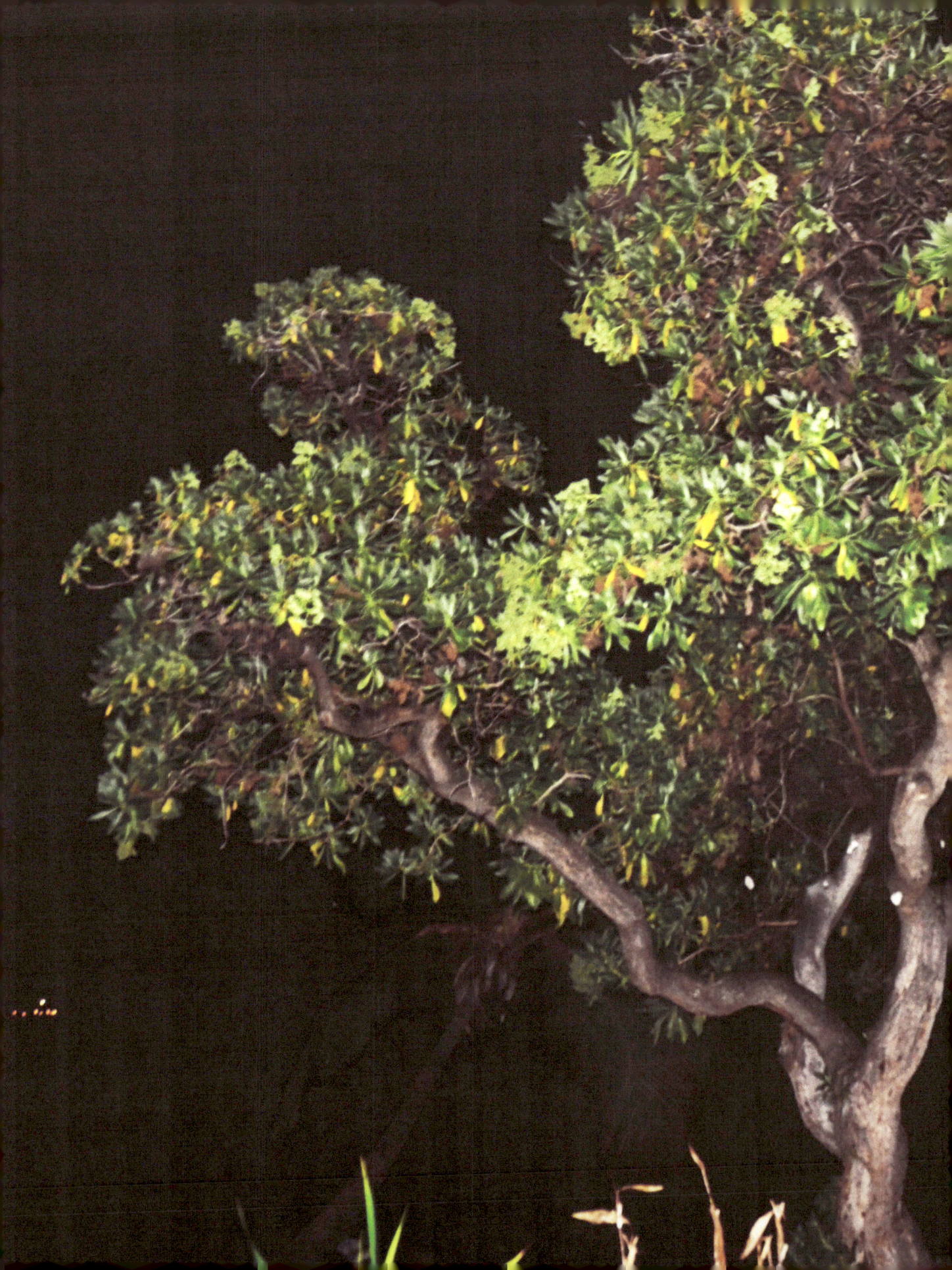

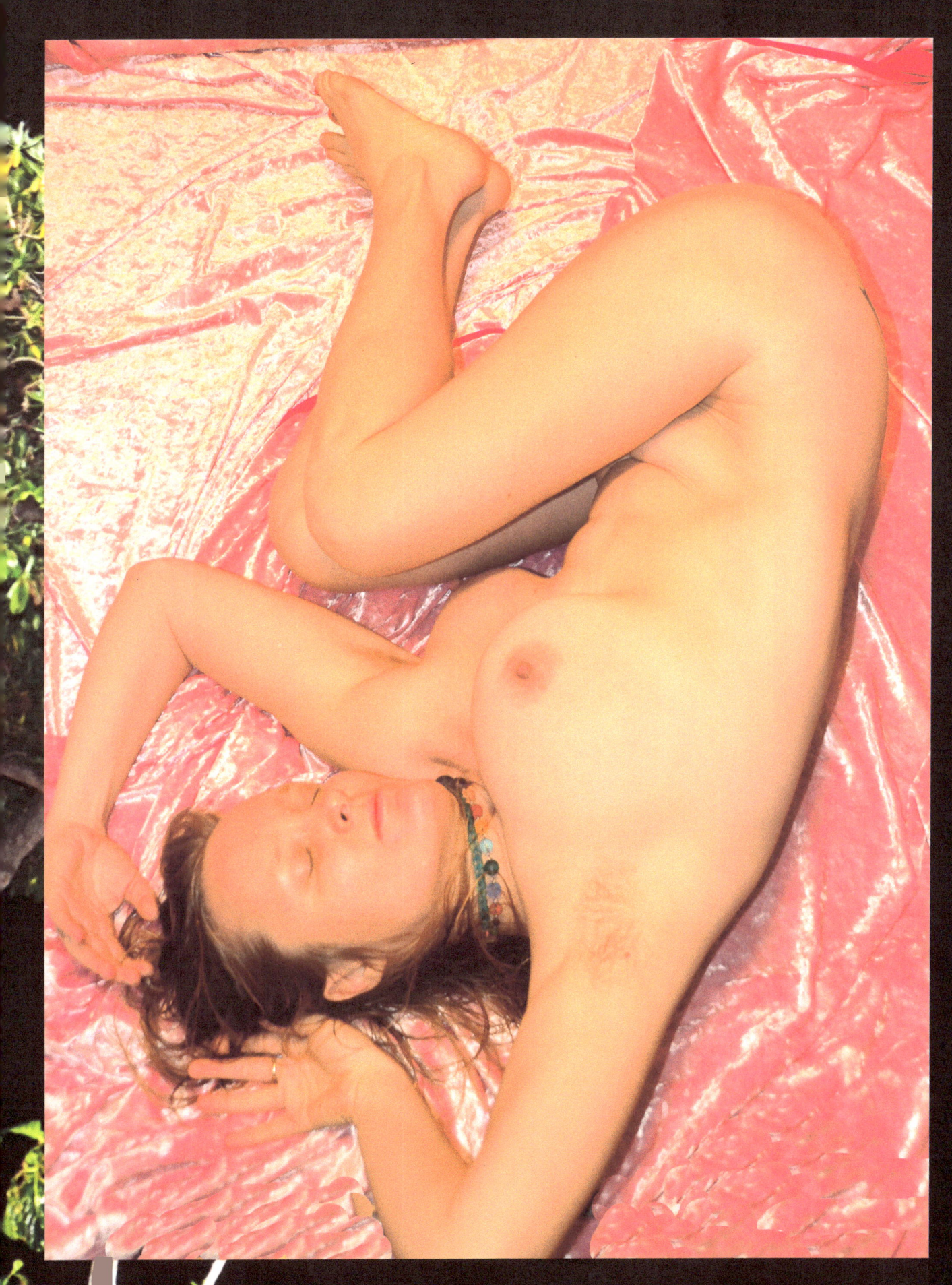

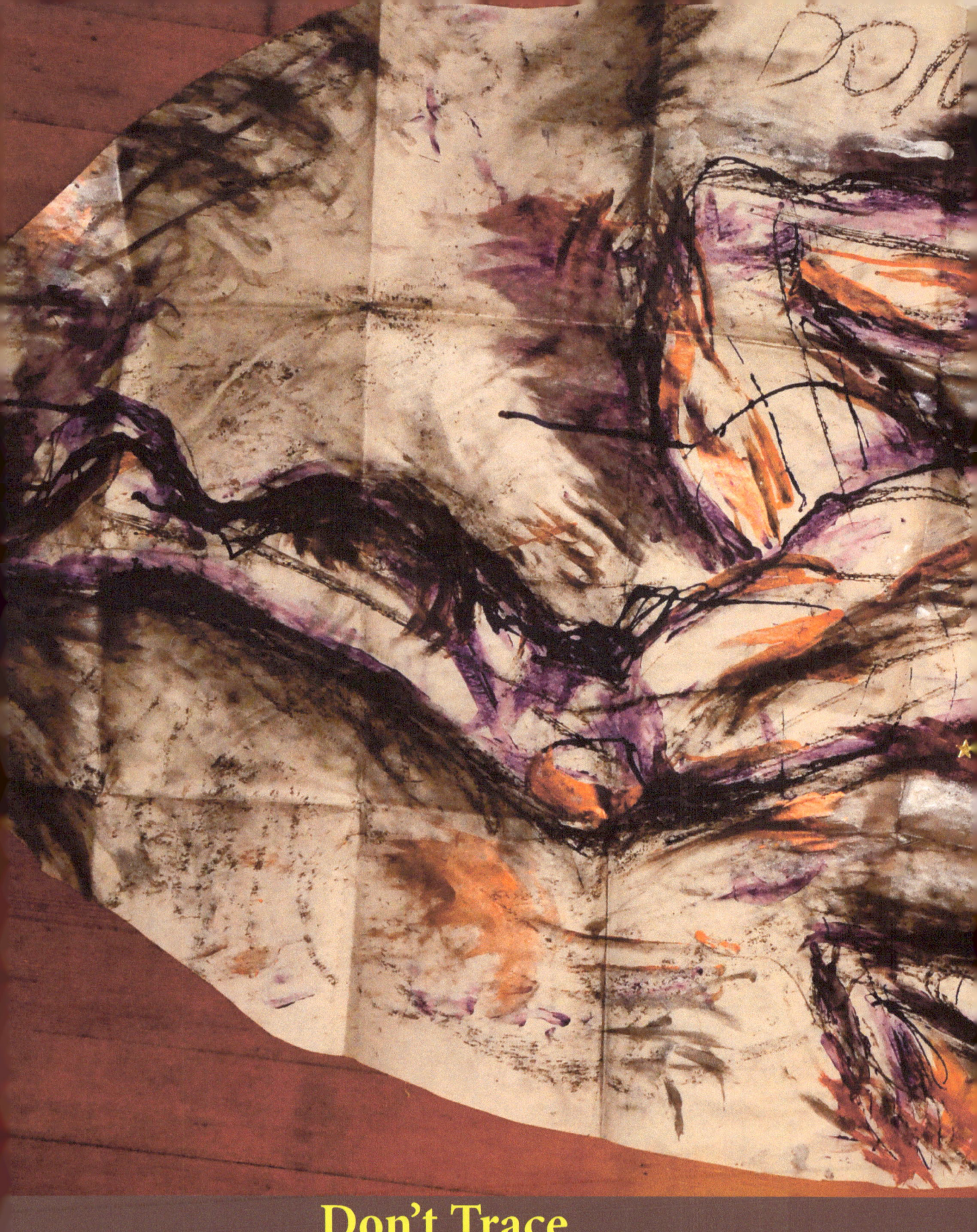

Don't Trace

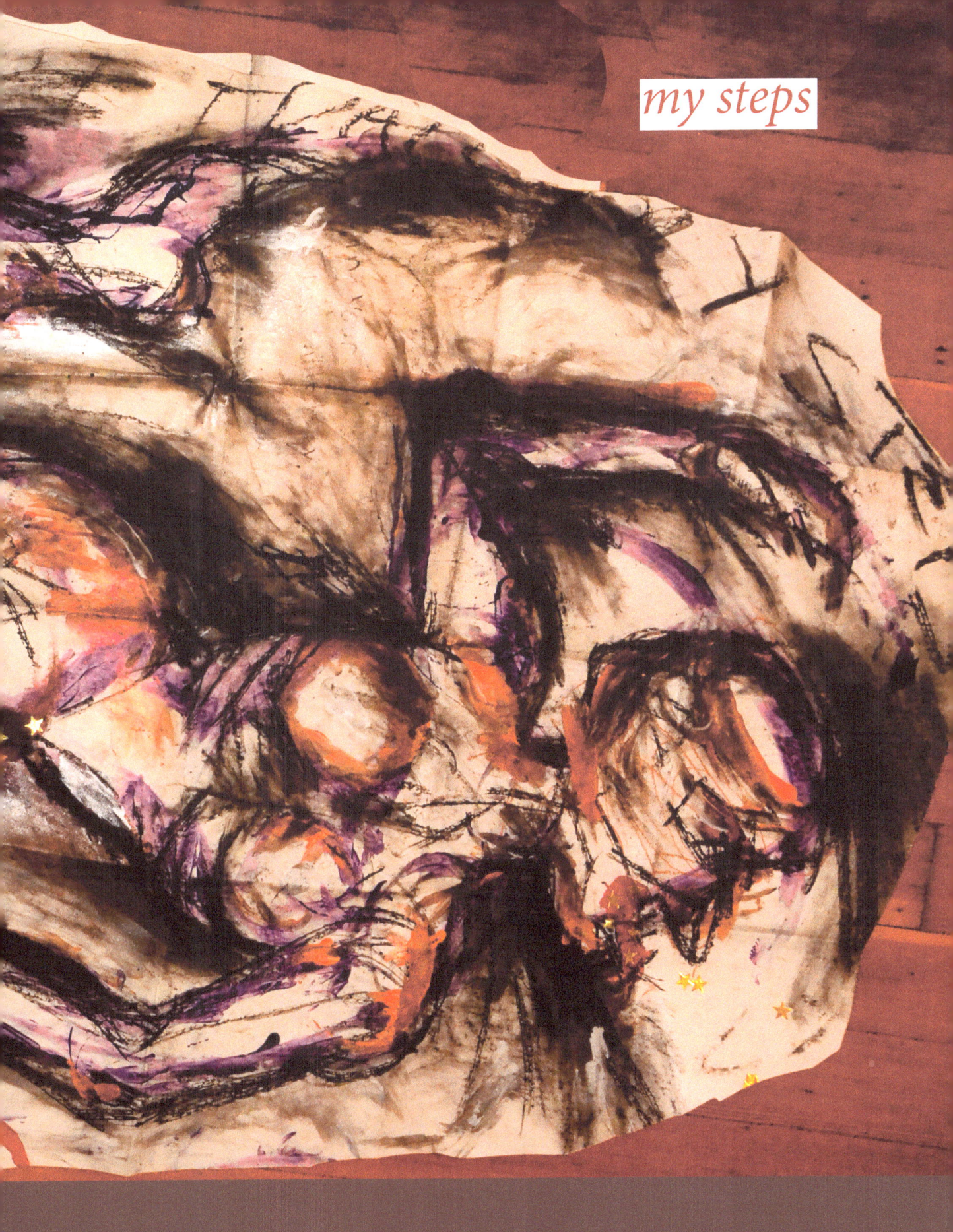

Uncovering layers of existence.....

ripping out my insides

shredding ideas of past
bursting into present
full force.

No chance to go back.
A choice everyday....to live or die.

The voice flows through
Spirit
travels its path.

We know where we are going.

Or do we?

Unveil ages, layers

CONFRONT YOUR TRUTH!!

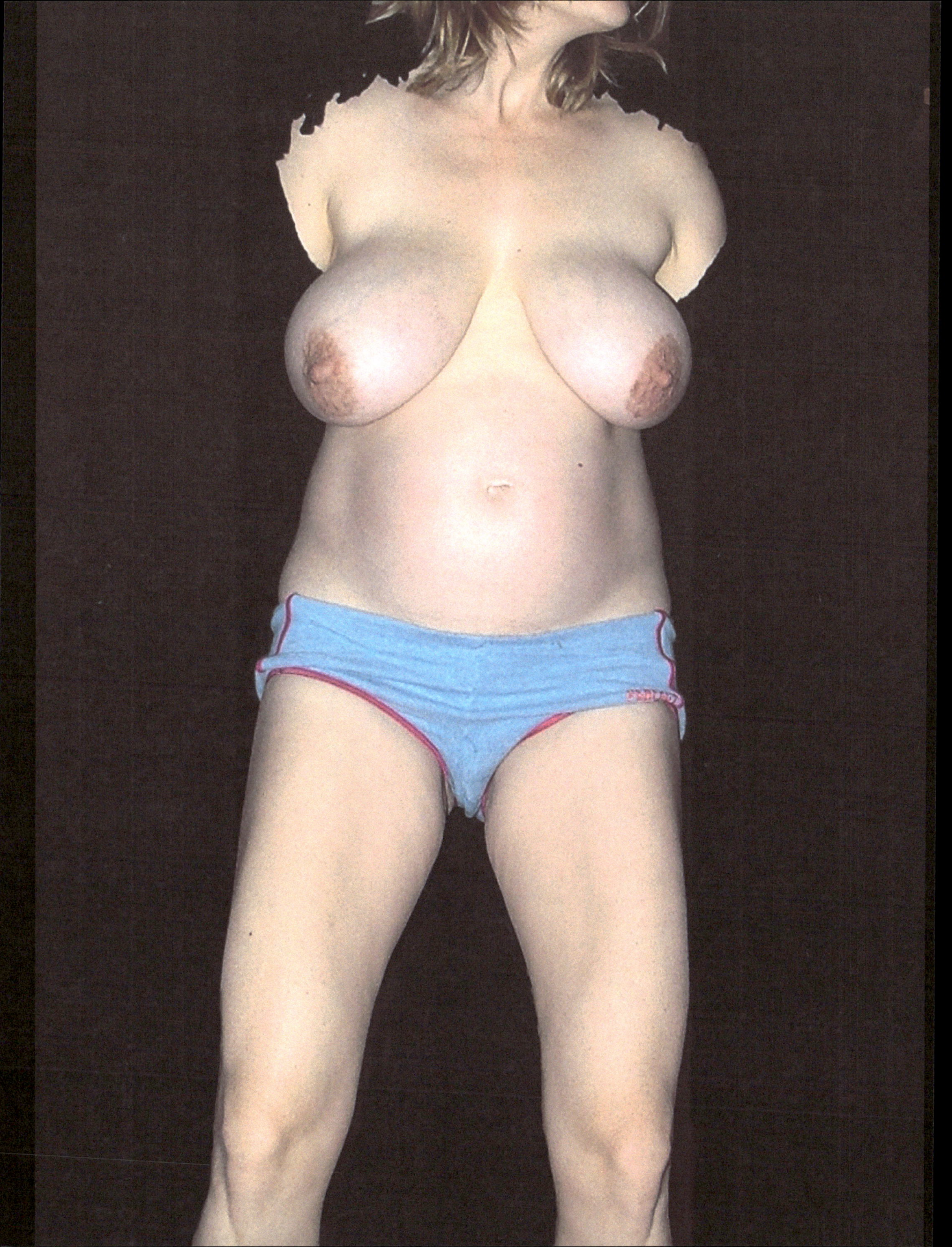

HAD A beautiful Day... Got a prescription for TOMAZAPAM that has helped a lot the last couple days. I feel groggy a bit during the day... but it has given me license to feel alive again after my melt down last week. I'm really not quite sure what happened ... too much? getting sick in her belly... her cavity getting treated? Gordon back at work after a week off taking such beautiful care of us? I just lit the candle for Tom again and opened his BOXES of Clothes. I was hoping to have one last little scent of him... But the clothes are a generic remembrance of his life and an ode to his philosophy... "TRAVEL LIGHTLY". HIS motto again+again. And so it would be so appropriate that these boxes of "things" are just that!? He never put much importance on STUFF! I just need to bring them to Goodwill.

2 things I
think ABOUT

① Tom's heart beat when I yelled his name
② The way his spirit left his BODY when I said by... HOW DEATH LOOKS.

April 22, 2010

I like the color of your pants I just don't like the ___ of them. The size is Fat legs.

Big Eye Sculpture

"AFTERLIFE"

(translation on following page)

Need to (study again :)

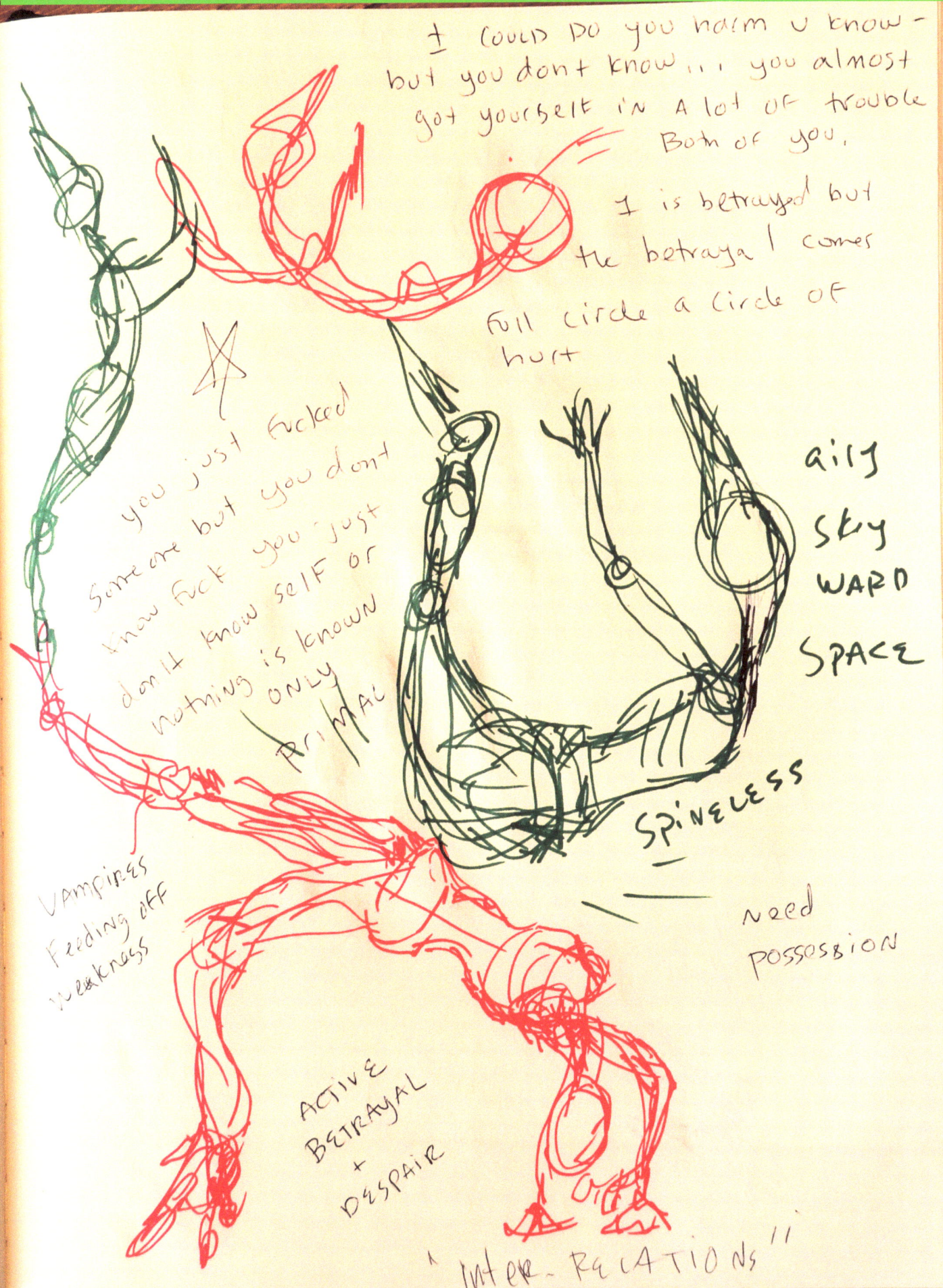

Beautiful day. A prescription for
tomazapam has helped the last
few days. I feel groggy. It's given me license
to feel alive again after what
happened... I lit a candle for my father
and opened his cardboard box of clothes,
hoping to have a scent of him. Only
generic rememberances of a lonely
nursing home life wafted out. An ode to
his philosphy: "travel lightly".
His motto again and again...

2 things i ponder:

1) My dad's heart beat when i yelled his
name

2) The way his spirit left his body when
I cried good bye minutes
before his death.

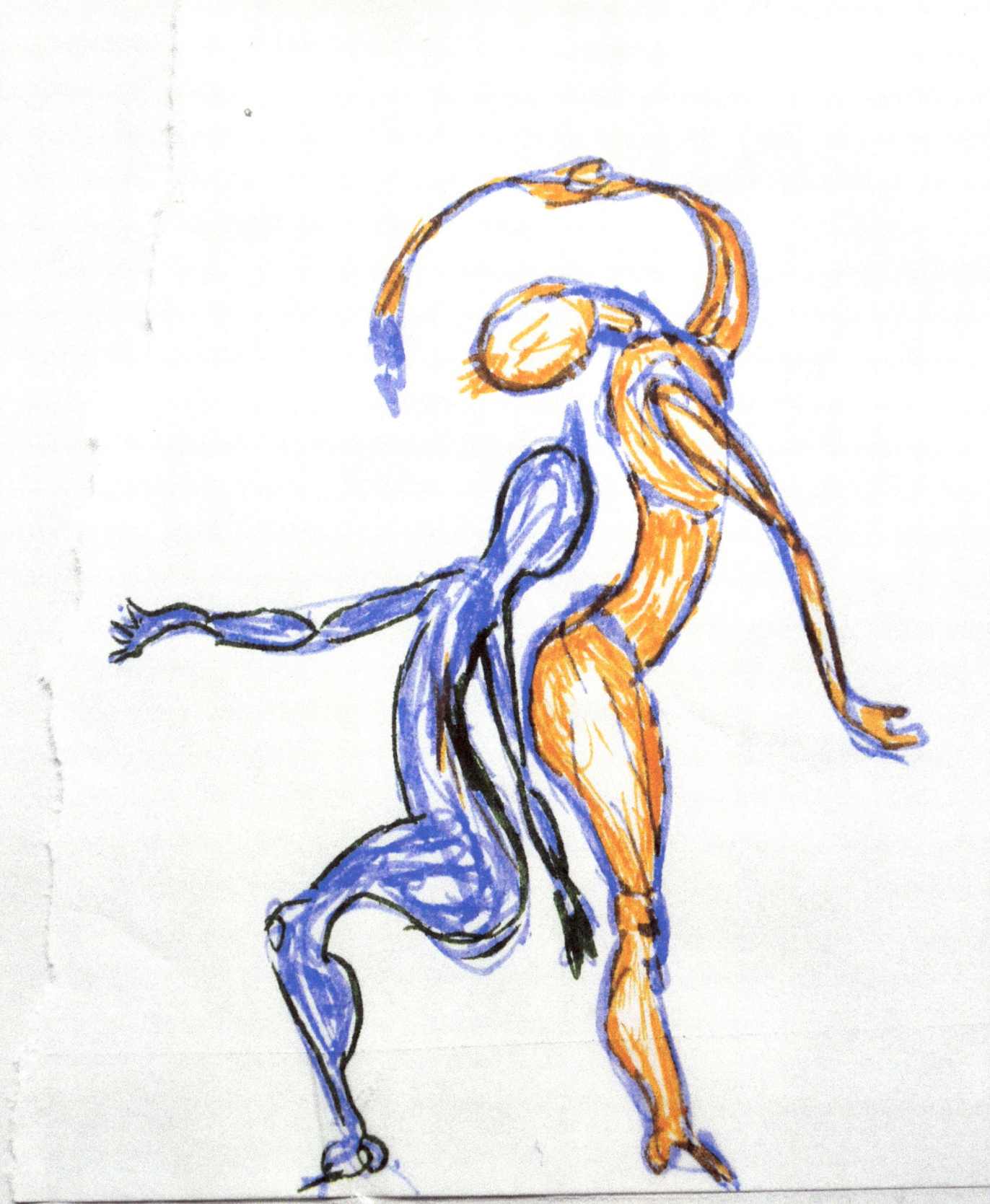

New stories

are created in the stew

of my bulging torso.

Out flushes a spirit

with an orbit to

unravel.

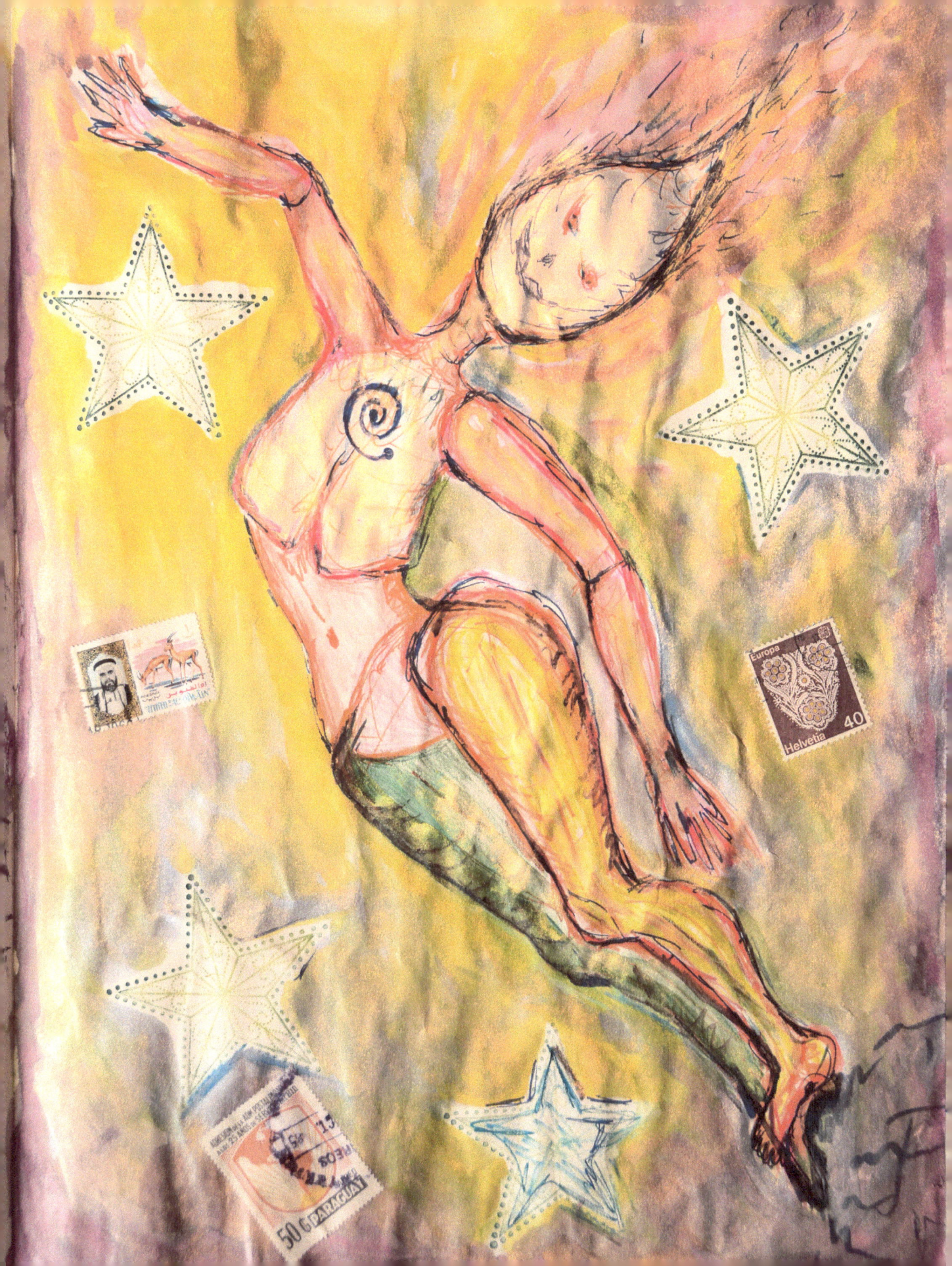

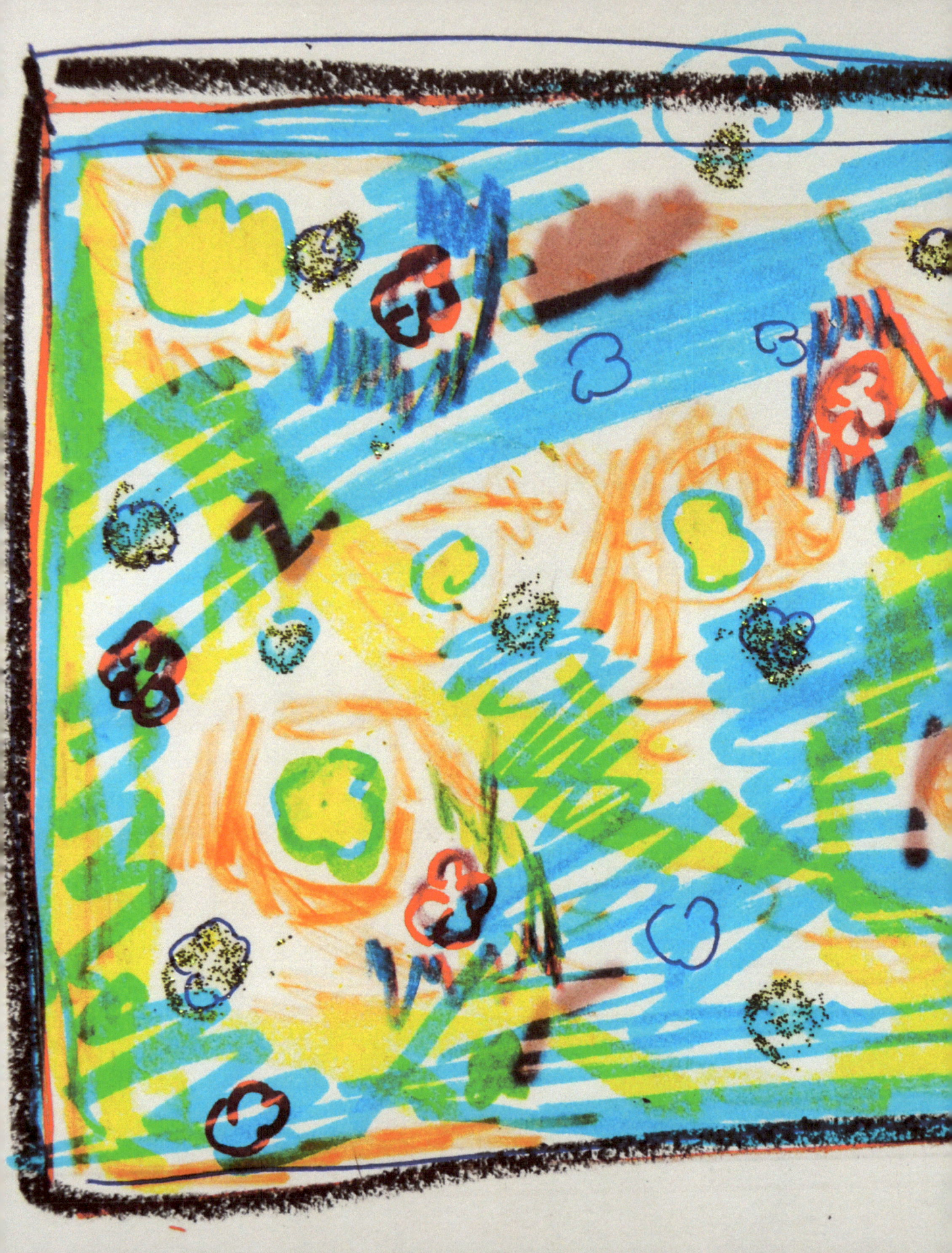

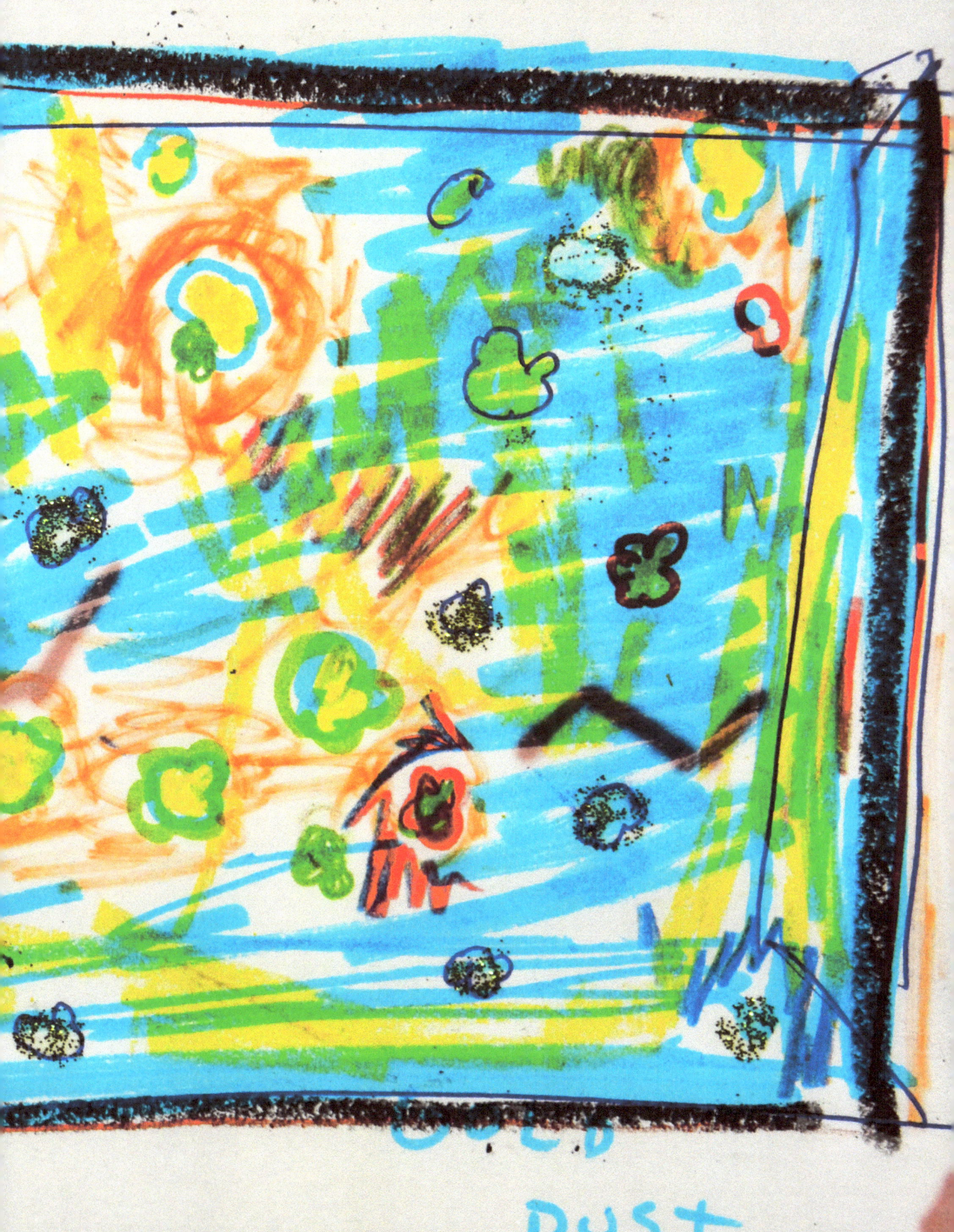

DUST

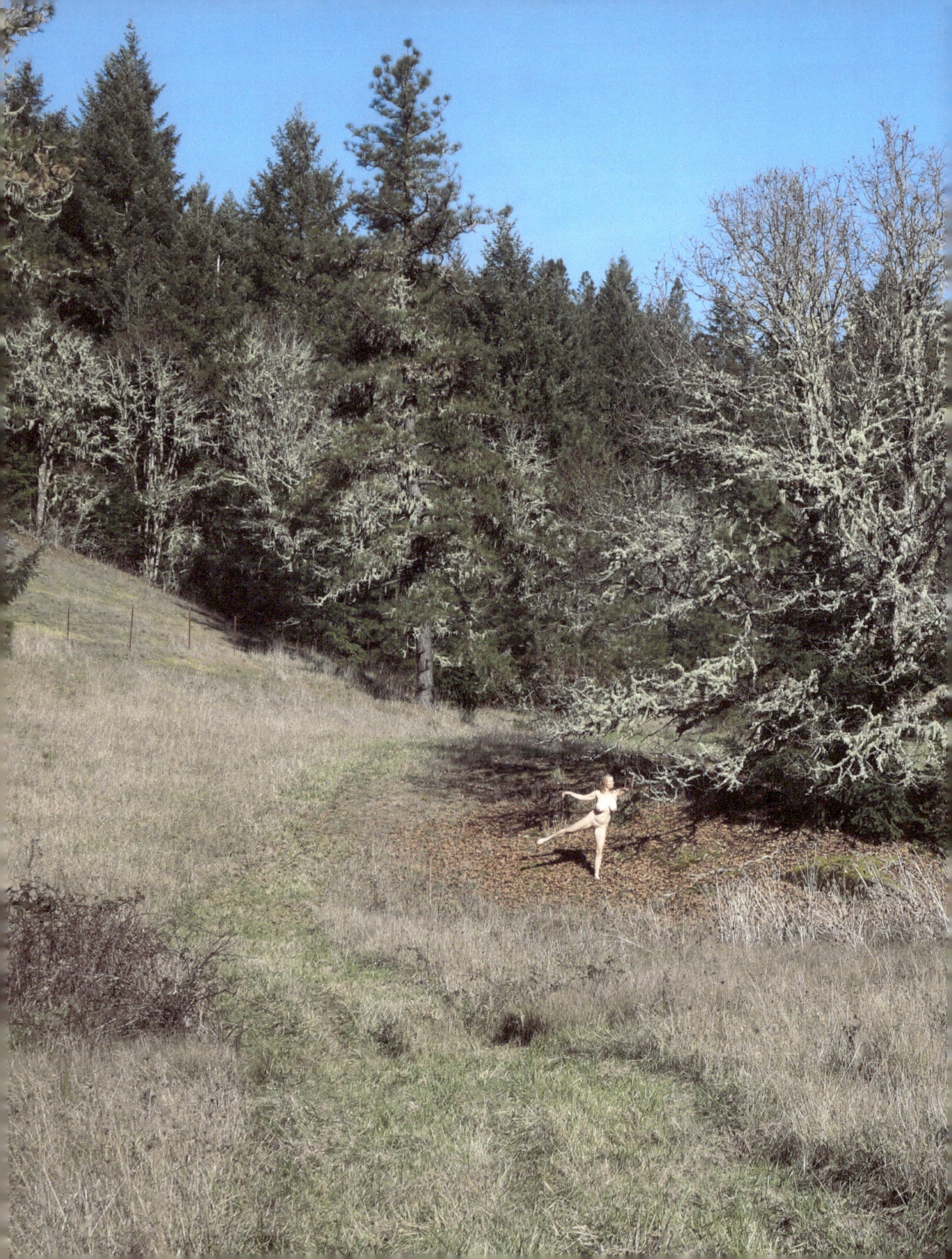

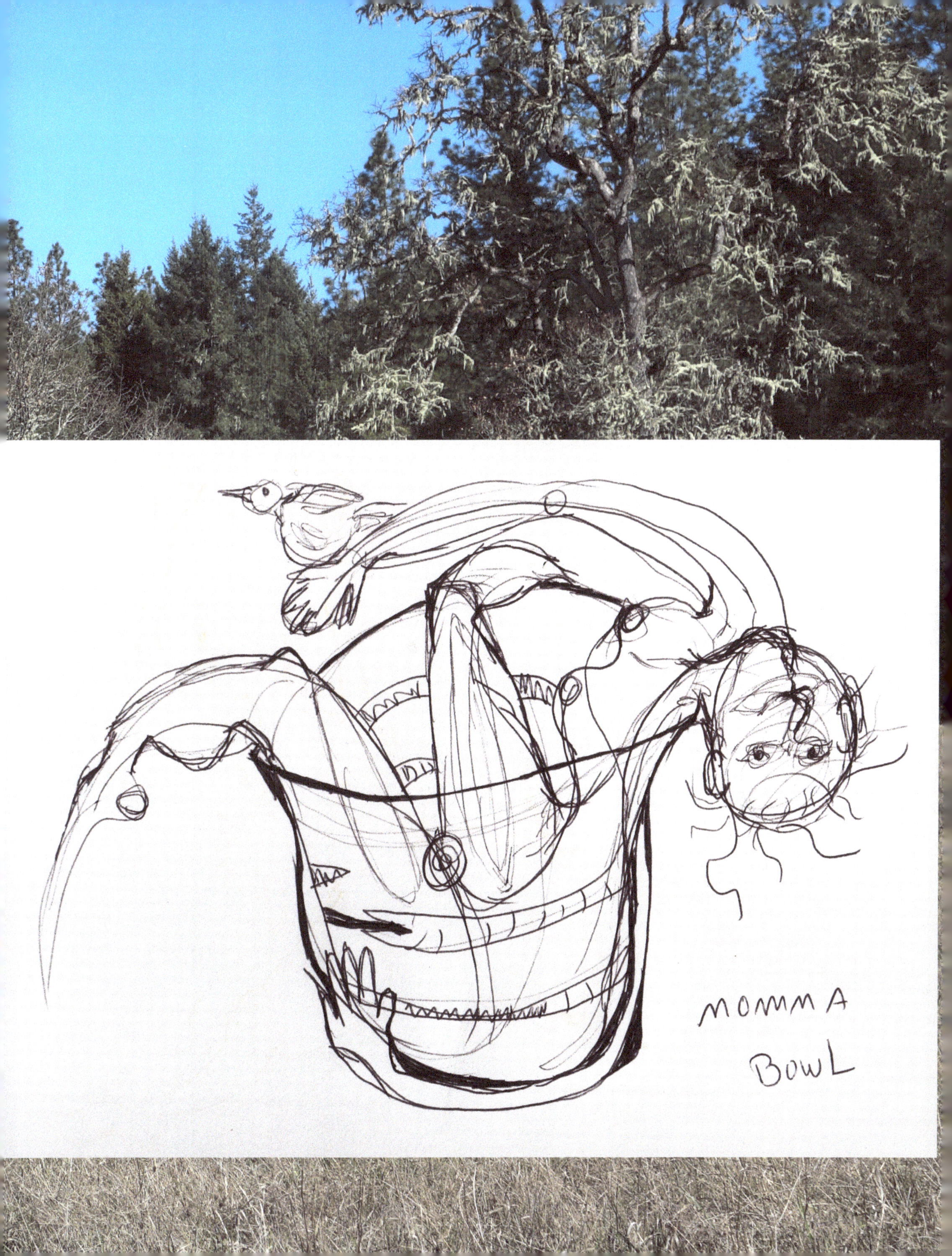

MOMMA
BOWL

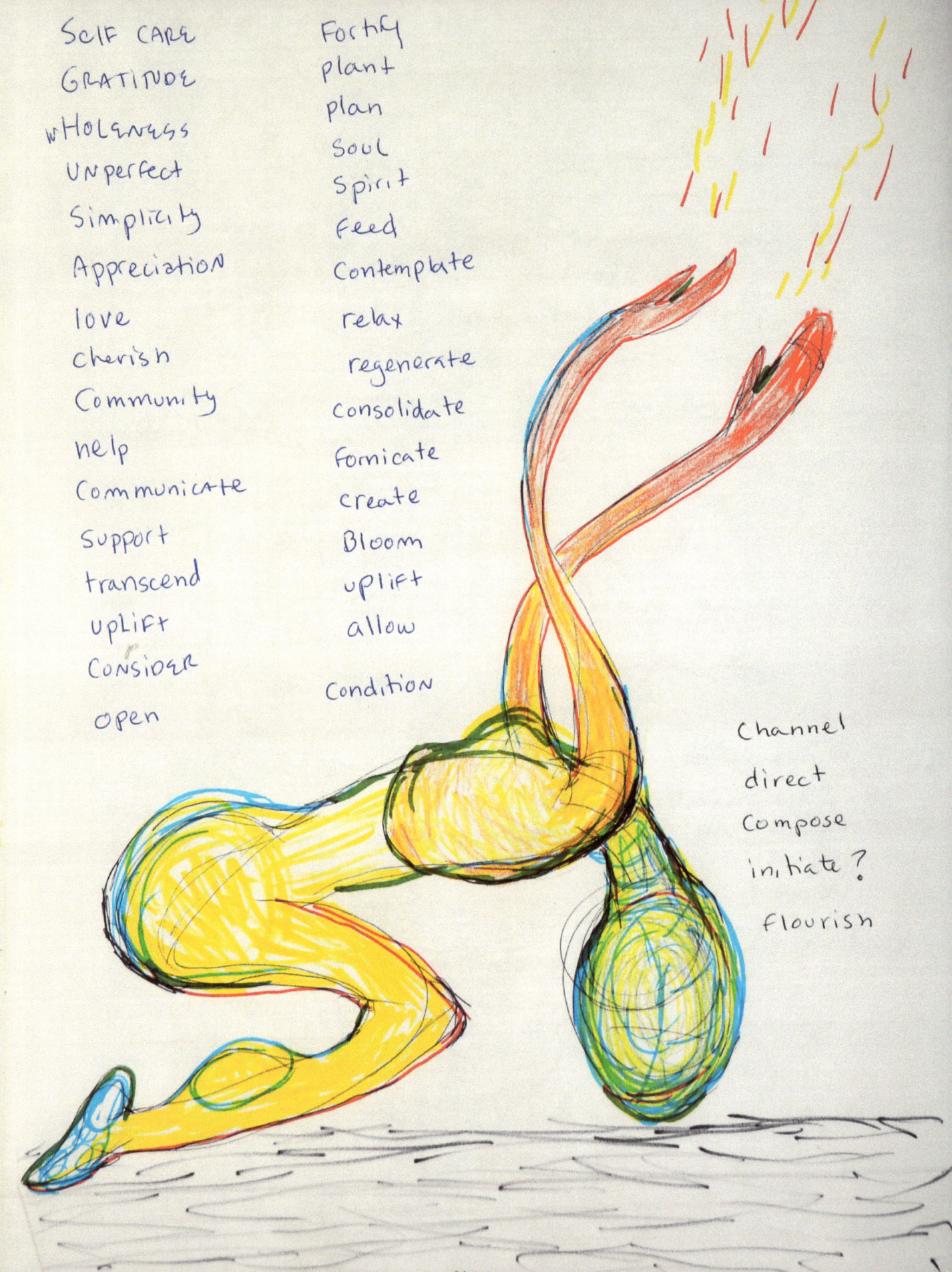

SELF CARE
GRATITUDE
WHOLENESS
UNPERFECT
Simplicity
Appreciation
love
cherish
Community
help
Communicate
Support
transcend
uplift
CONSIDER
open

Fortify
plant
plan
Soul
Spirit
Feed
Contemplate
relax
regenerate
consolidate
Fornicate
create
Bloom
uplift
allow

Condition

Channel
direct
Compose
initiate?
Flourish

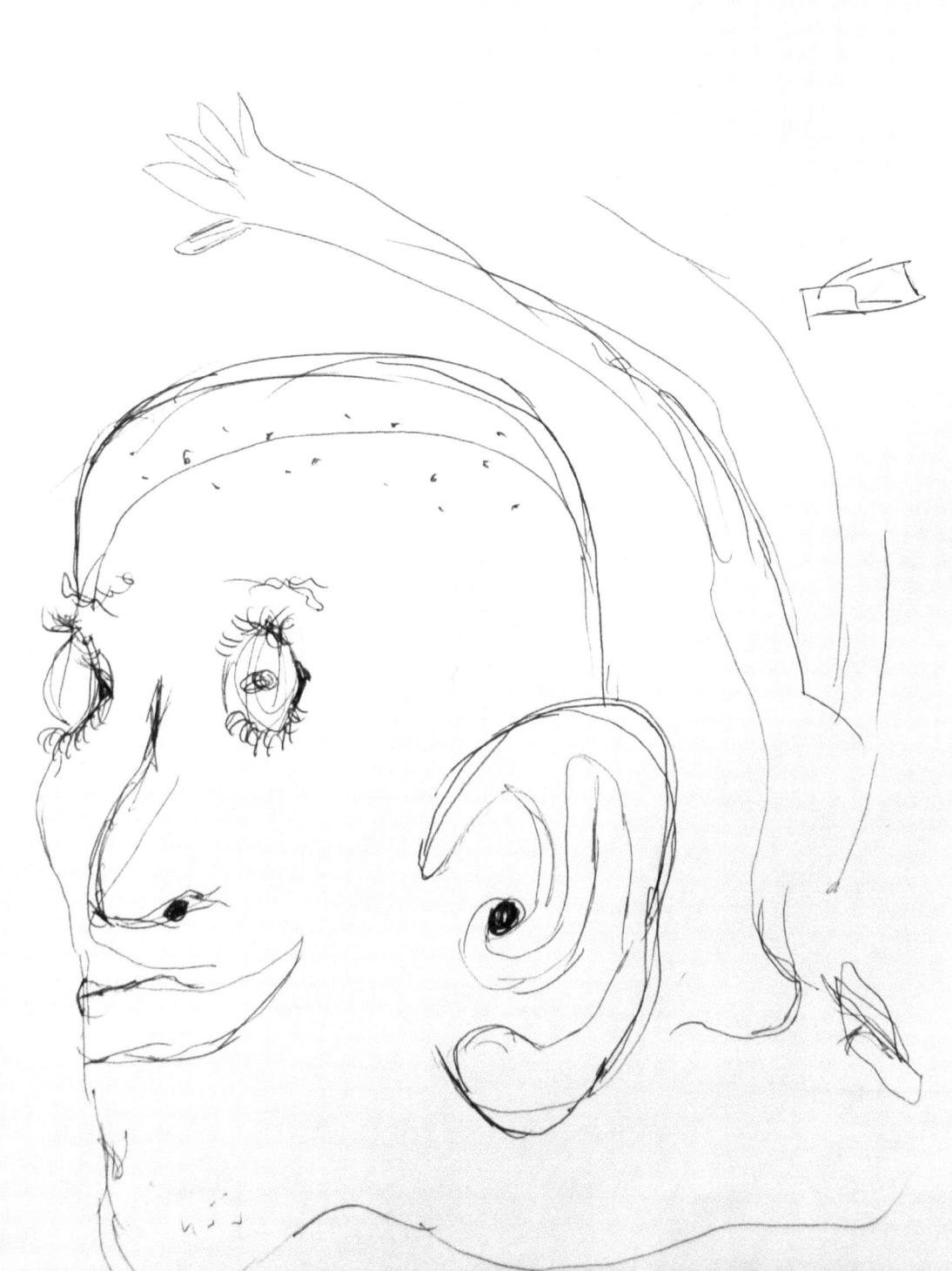

LARGE SCULPTURE ORGANIC BODIES

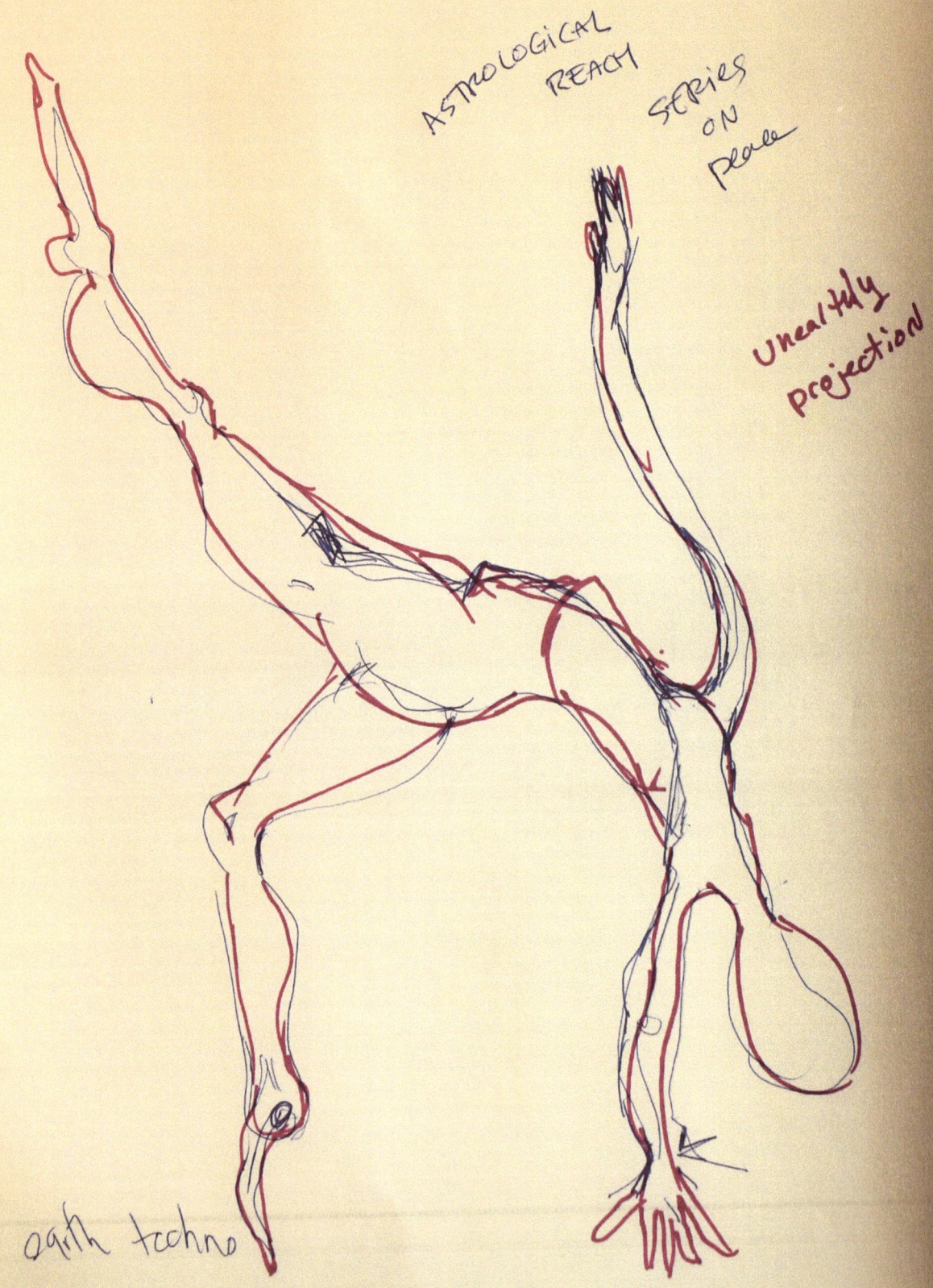

ASTROLOGICAL
REACH

SERIES
ON
Peace

unearthly
projection

a9th techno

DIRECTION

Talking + having passion for ART gives service + importance.

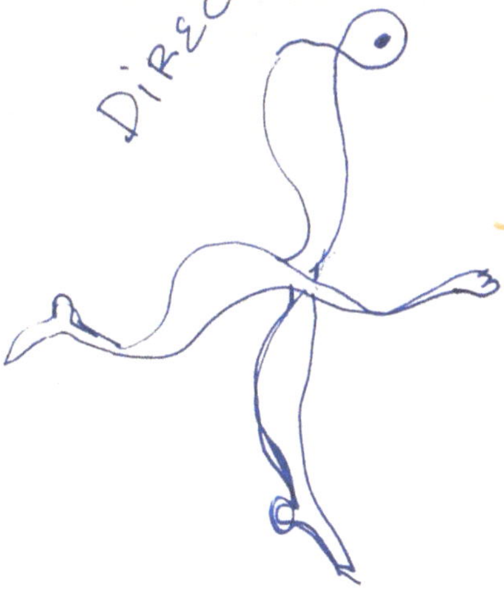

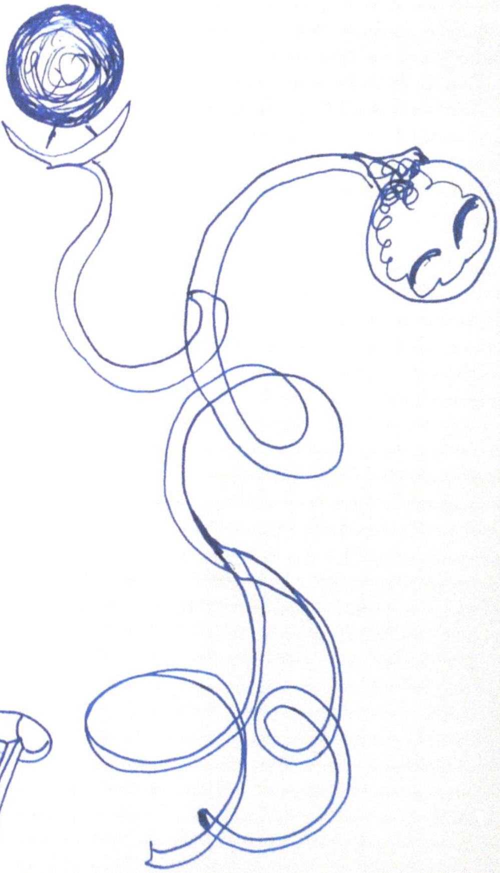

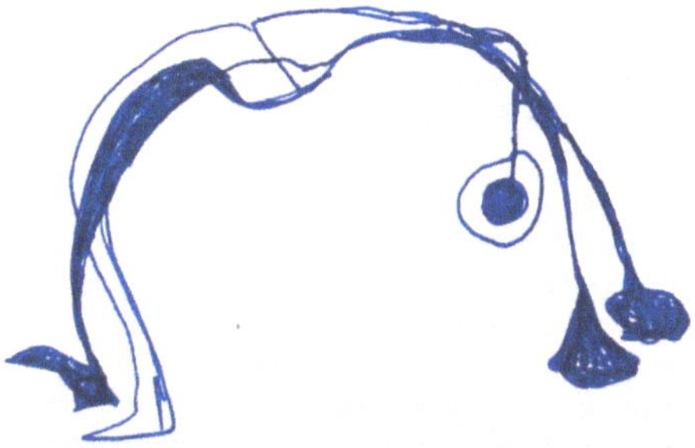

insect VS. MAN

Flowering

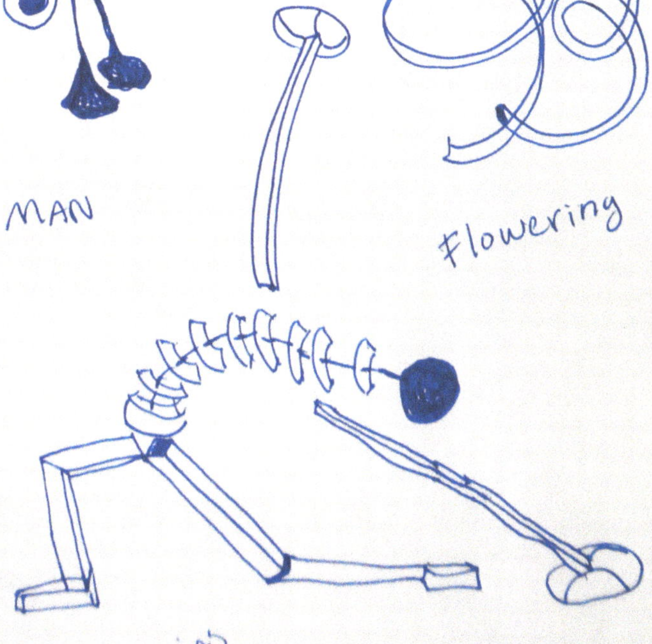

trying to emote

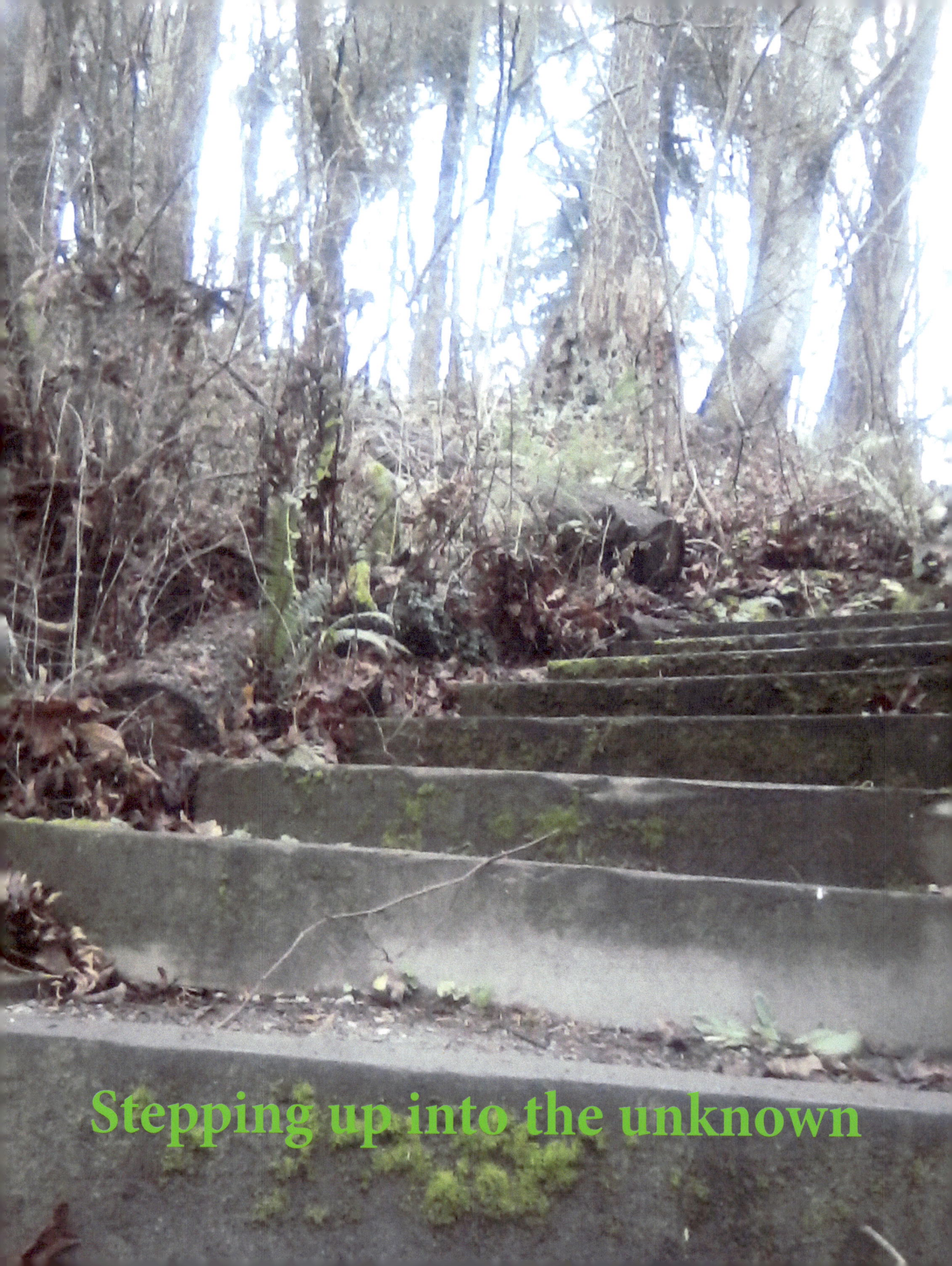

Stepping up into the unknown

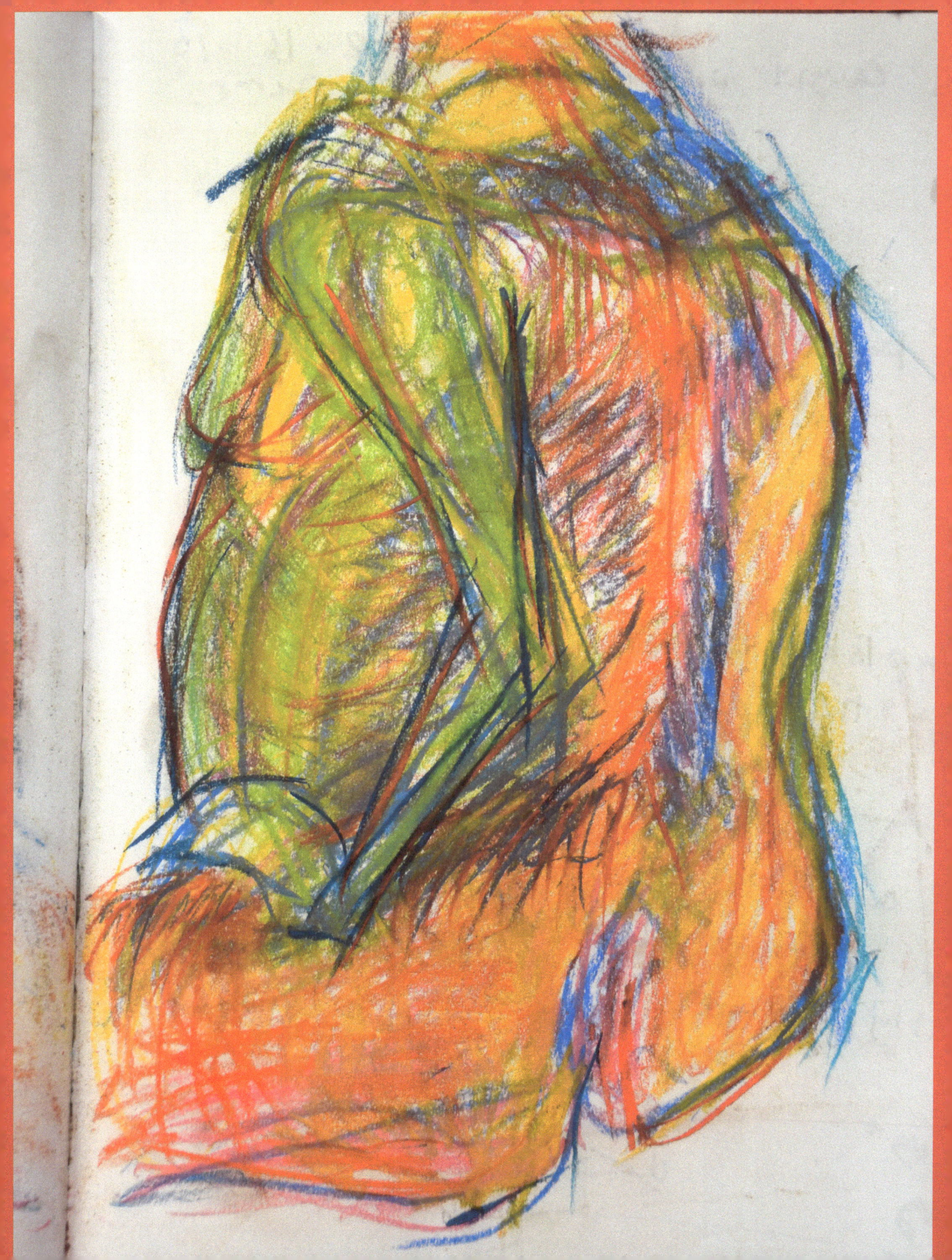

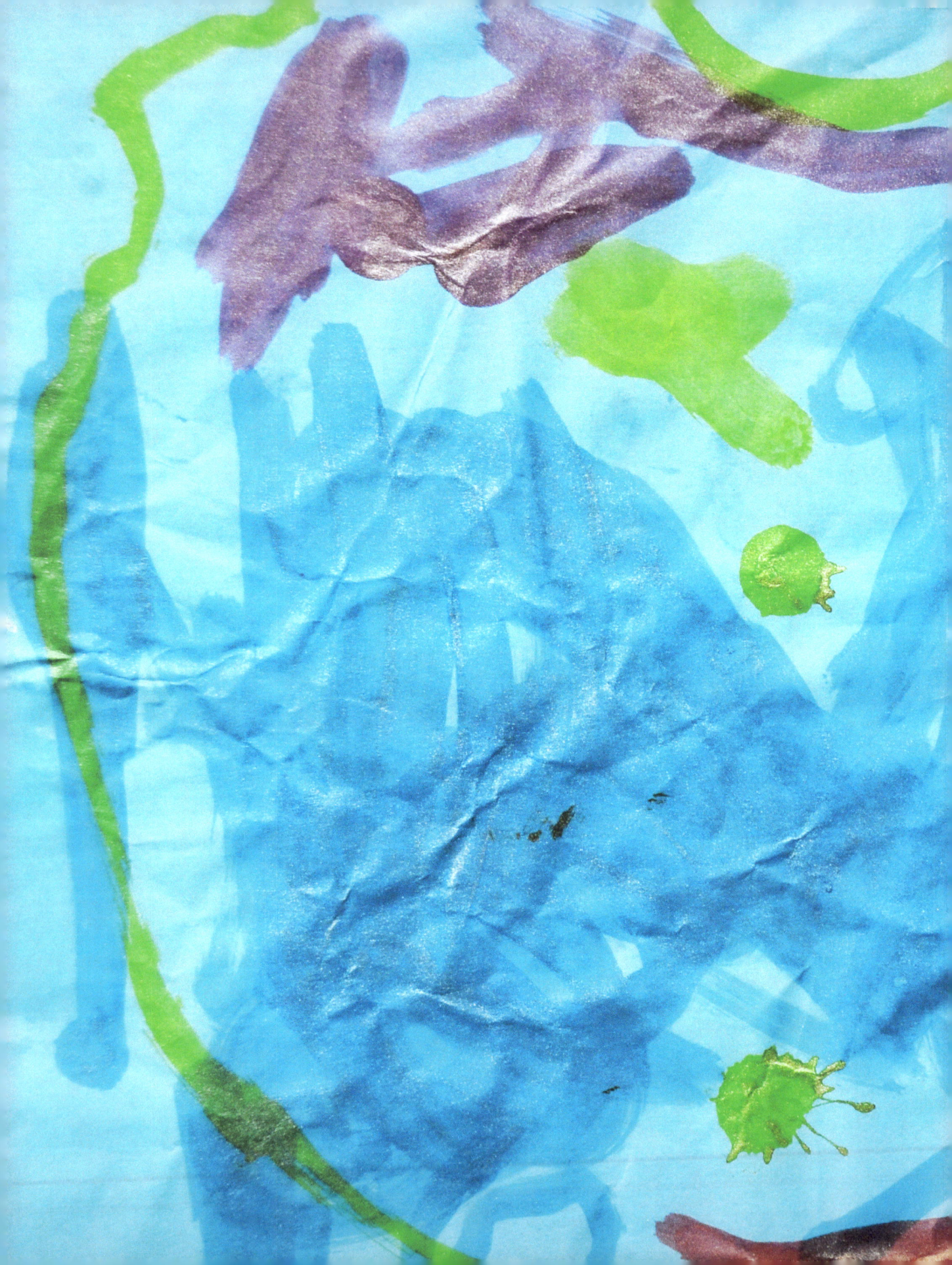

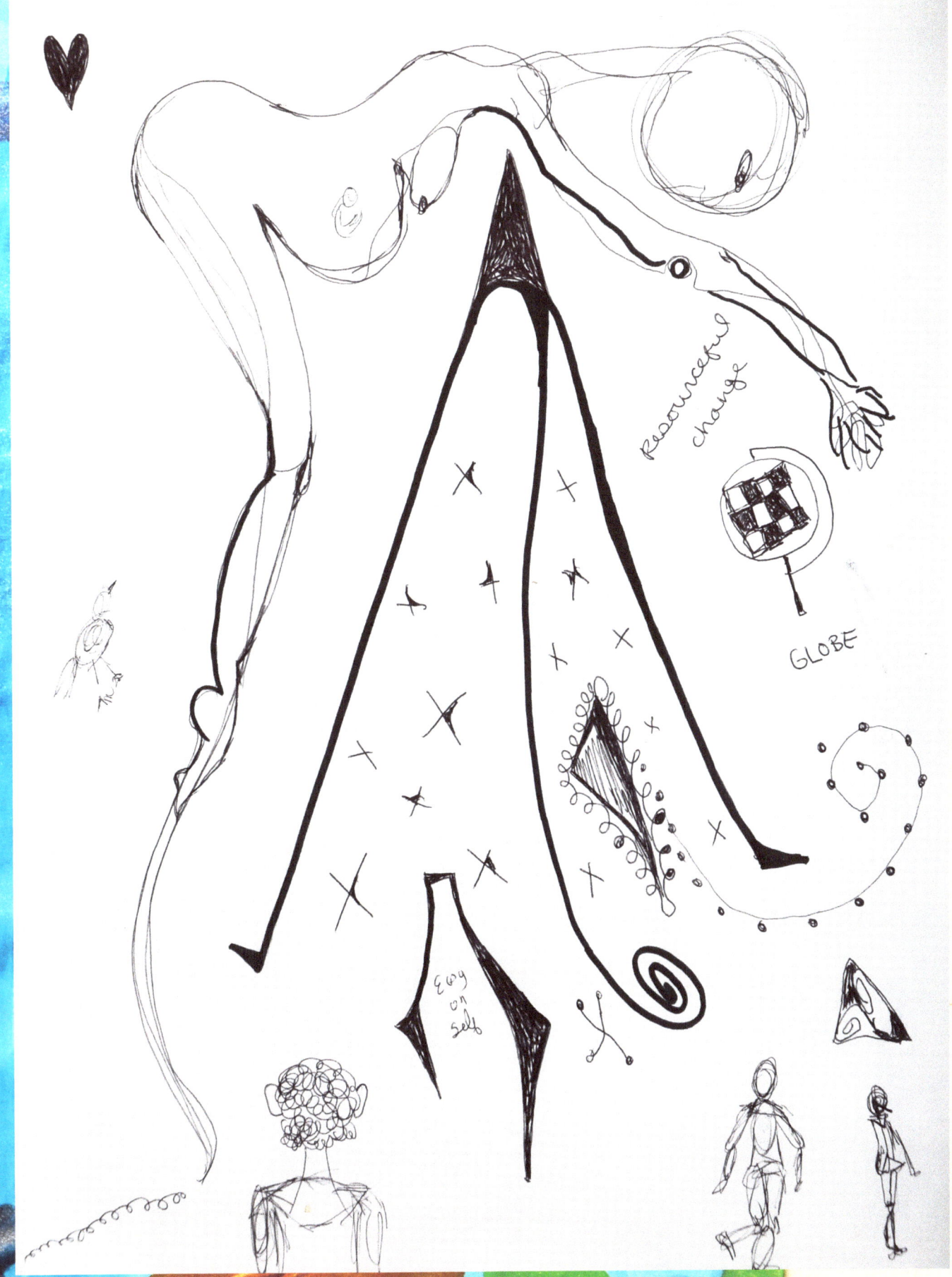

The process is underestimated.
It is torture...
Confronting reality
versus expectation; fantasy.
To cross the hurdle of
everything. Its life, its death,
it is becoming a drunkard,
heroine addict or song bird.
Not right or wrong...
an immediate choice.
Conscious or
predestined?

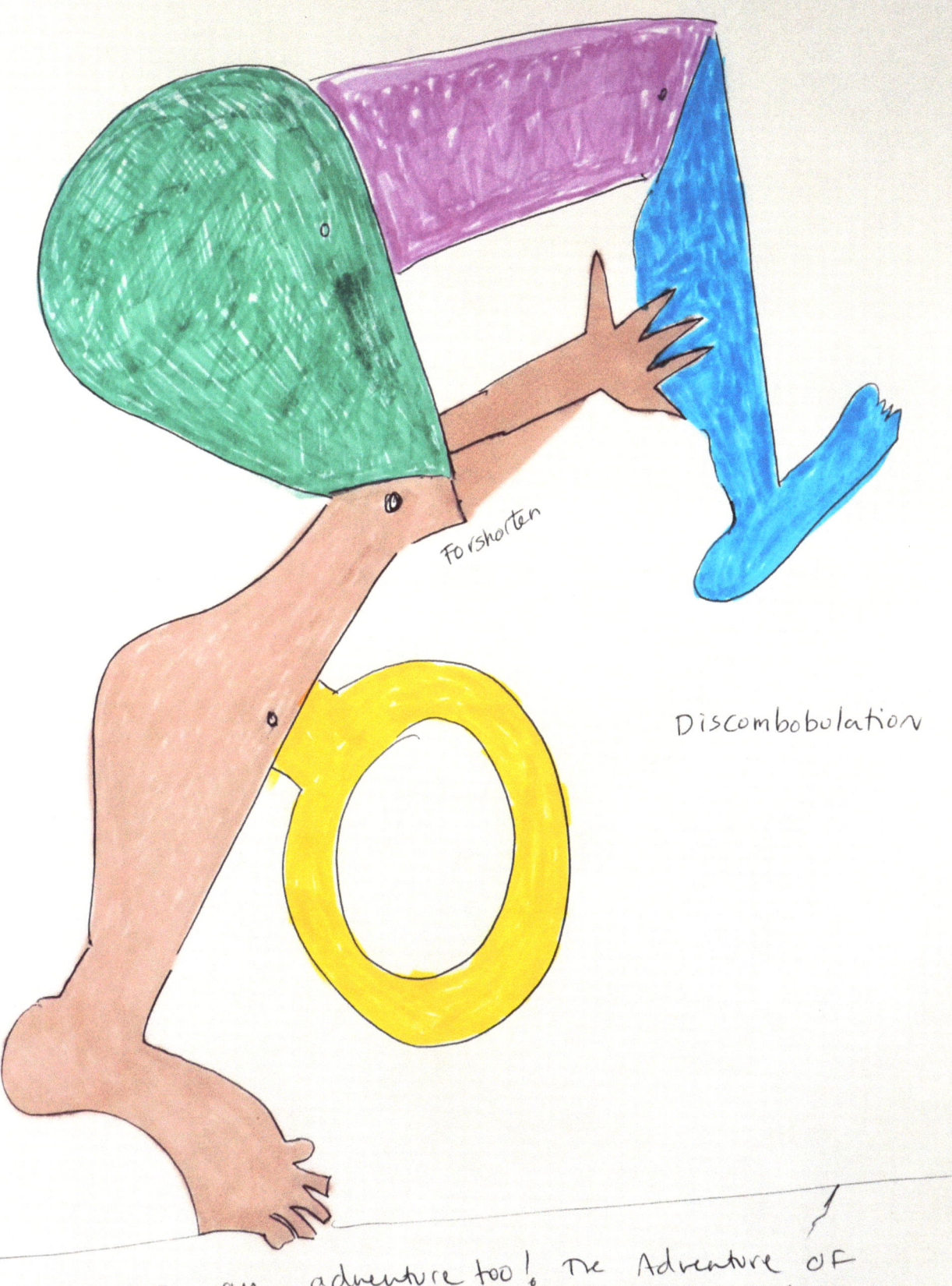

Forshorten

Discombobulation

well, I am on an adventure too!. The Adventure of mommyhood in 2011! I have a 6 year old el/luv and a body that wont sleep ... how endearing.

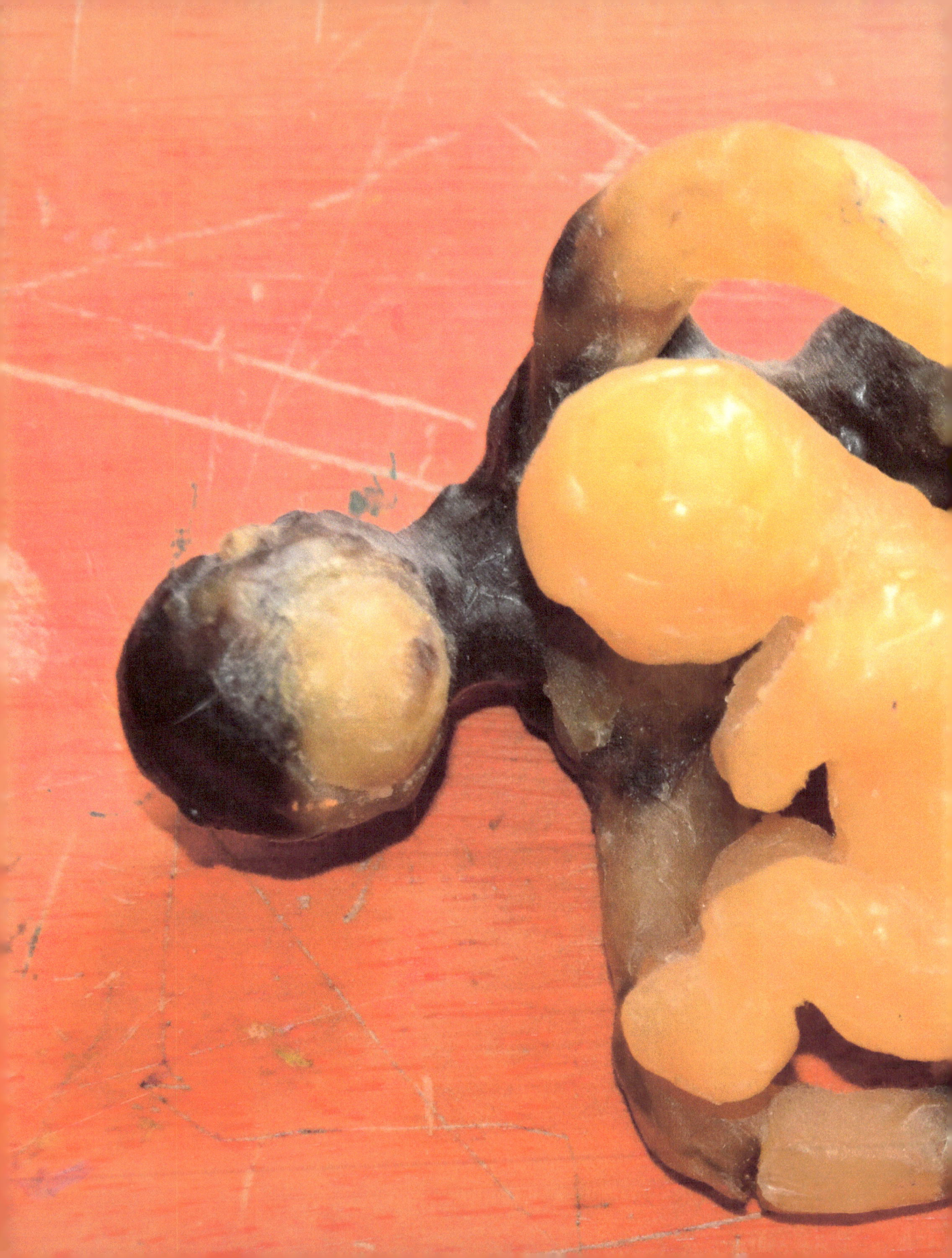

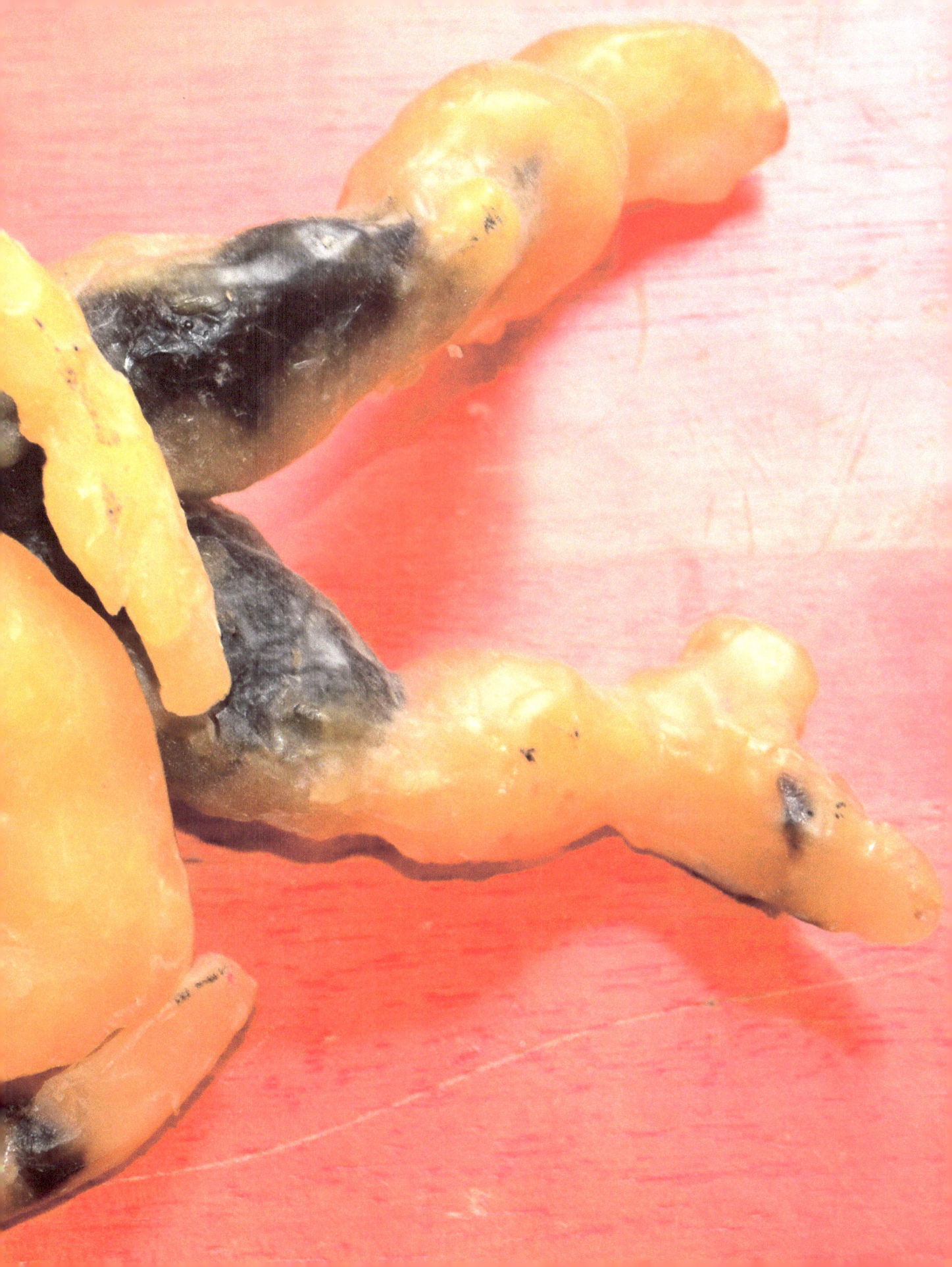

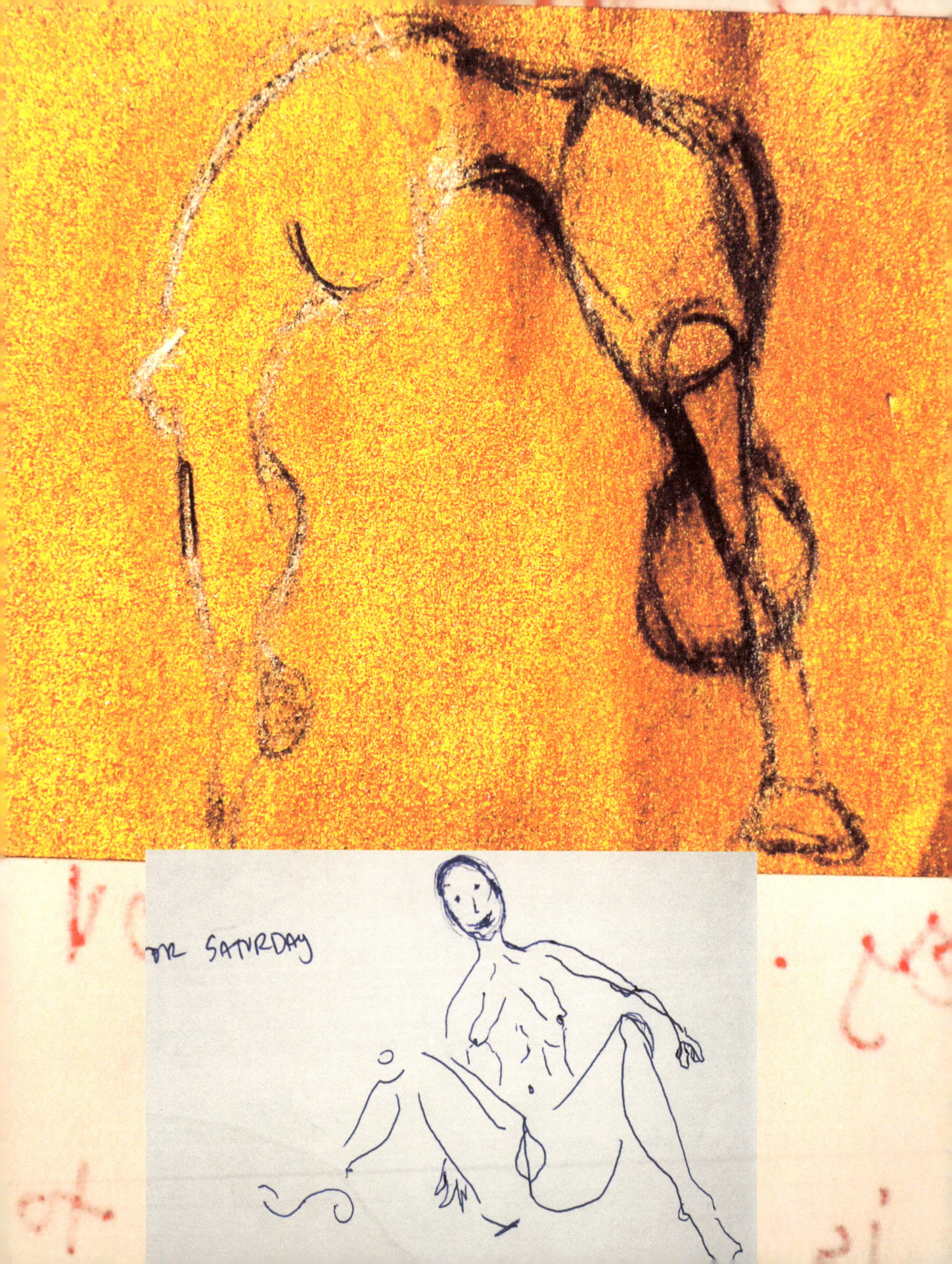

OR SATURDAY

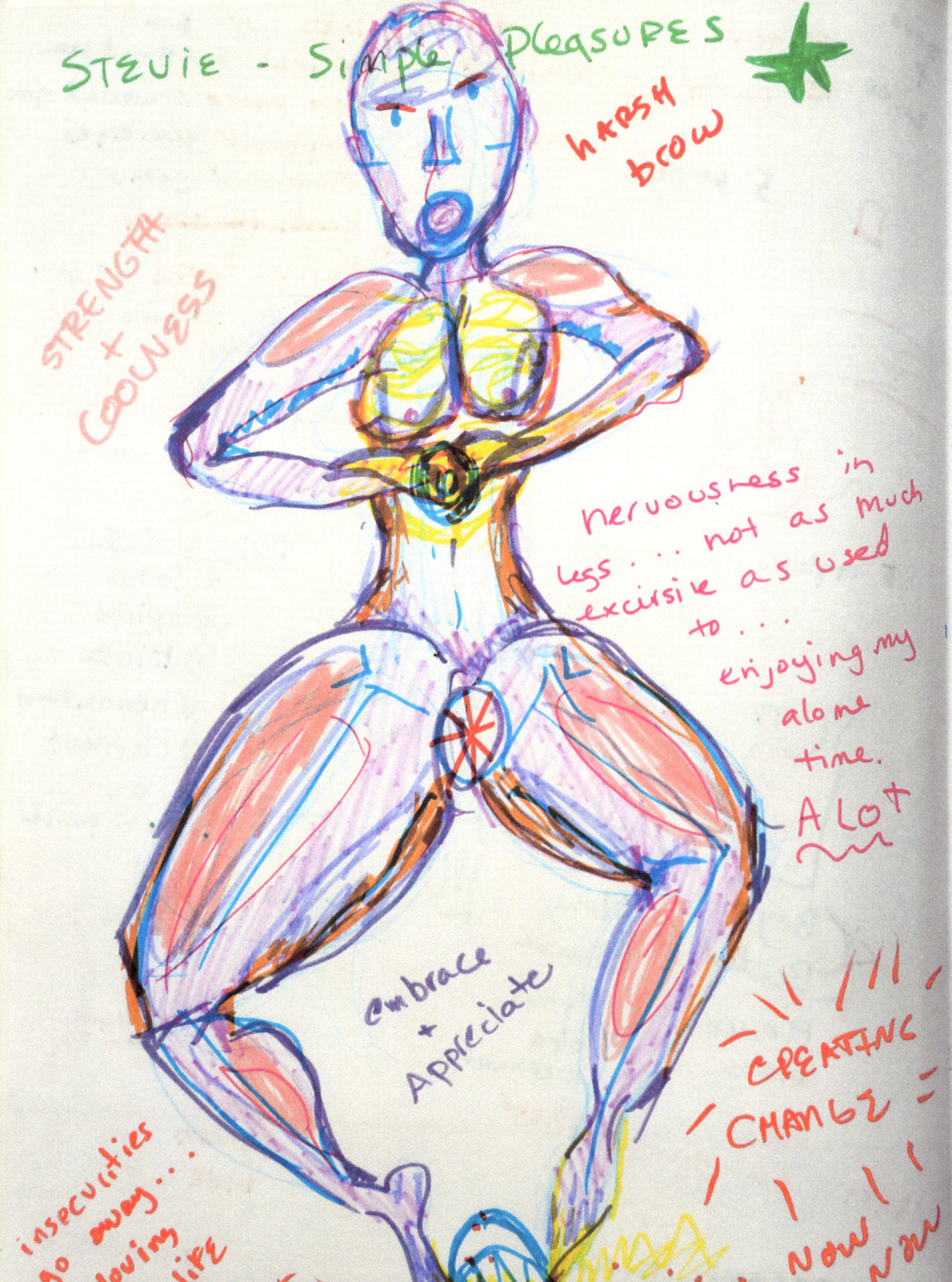

I already thought that and will have time to rest.

10-20-2011   1 A.M.

Painting class ... relax ...
All ok.   love peace ...

BRAIN FOG THE DREAM BOY

like a
shoe

me Comorrow, how to Cre

work togeth
teachig Pe
plans?

Ch

drawing . . . walk to school
o , CAlm.

DRAWing of

Y

New Friend

Brain Fog
again. ex

SPACe
Ship
TRee

LEG

when I DON'T

AGe is A ro
keeping bra

TRee of
Life Spirit

I already
Now is the

FIGHTING WITH

ISOLATE

GRATIUDE

PLANNING

DEAREST

HOLD

STRENGTH

FORTINDE

HOLD

FOUNDATION

ENVELOPE

PLACEMENT

STEADY

YOURSELF

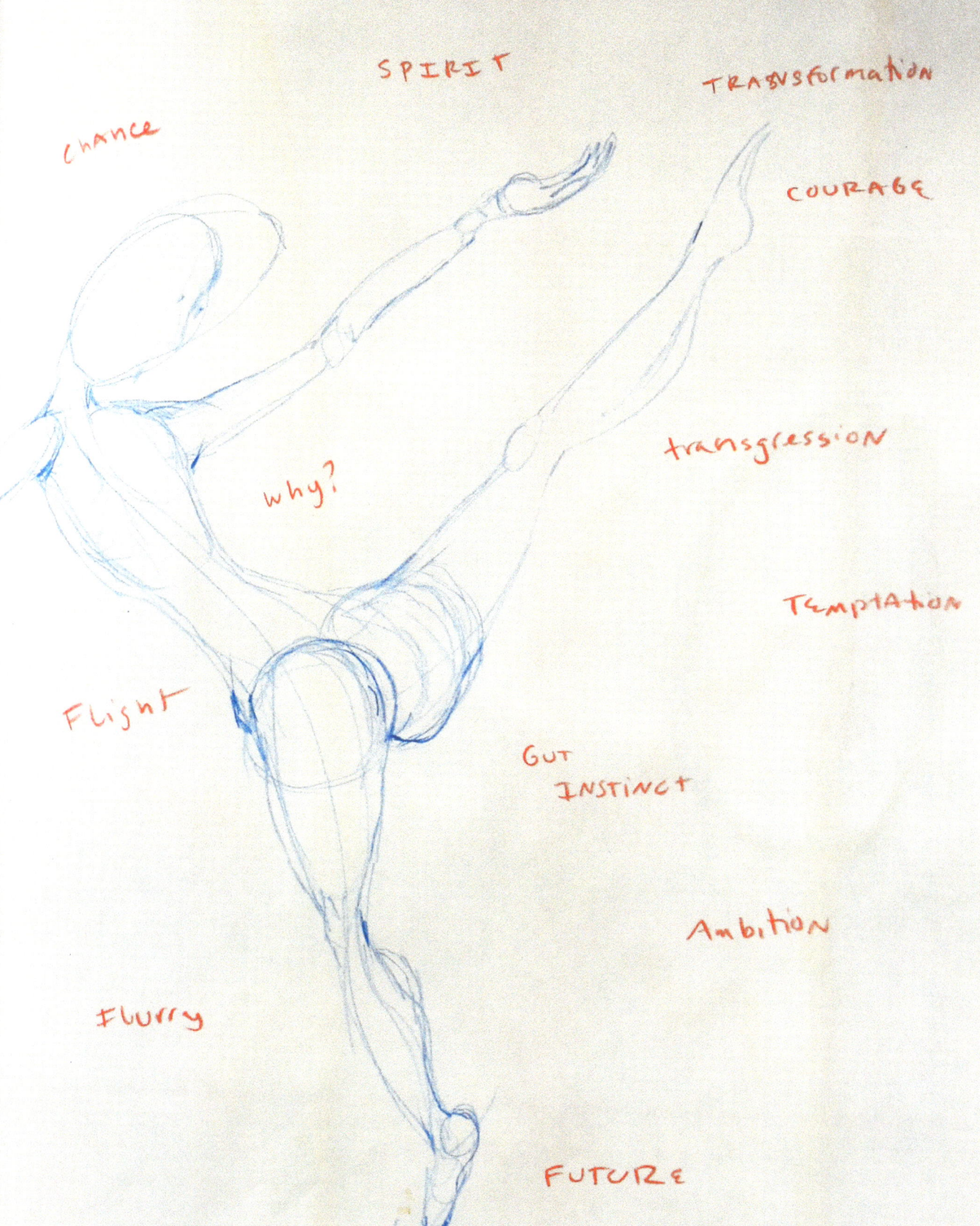

SPIRIT

TRANSFORMATION

Chance

COURAGE

transgression

why?

TEMPTATION

Flight

GUT
INSTINCT

Ambition

Flurry

FUTURE

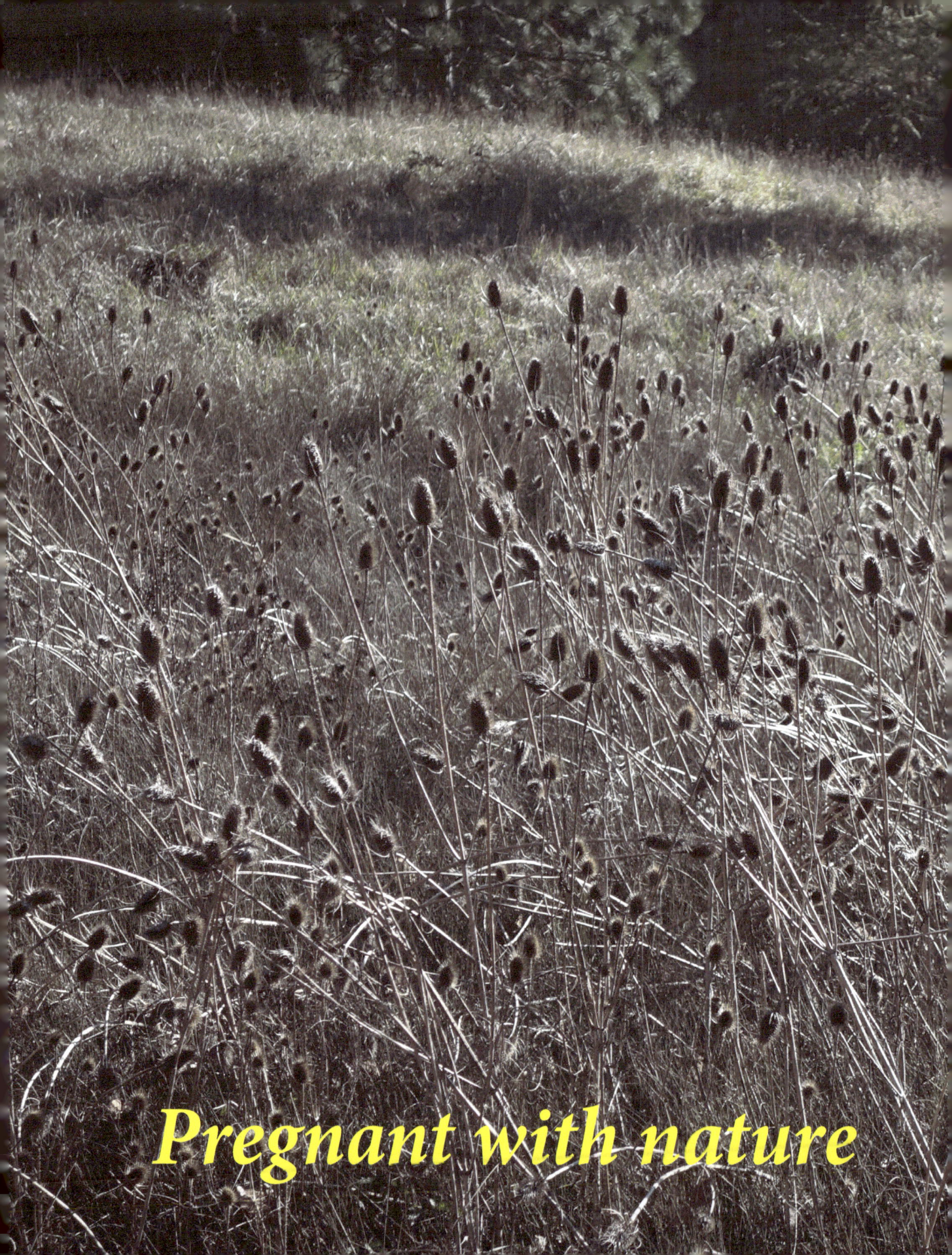

Pregnant with nature

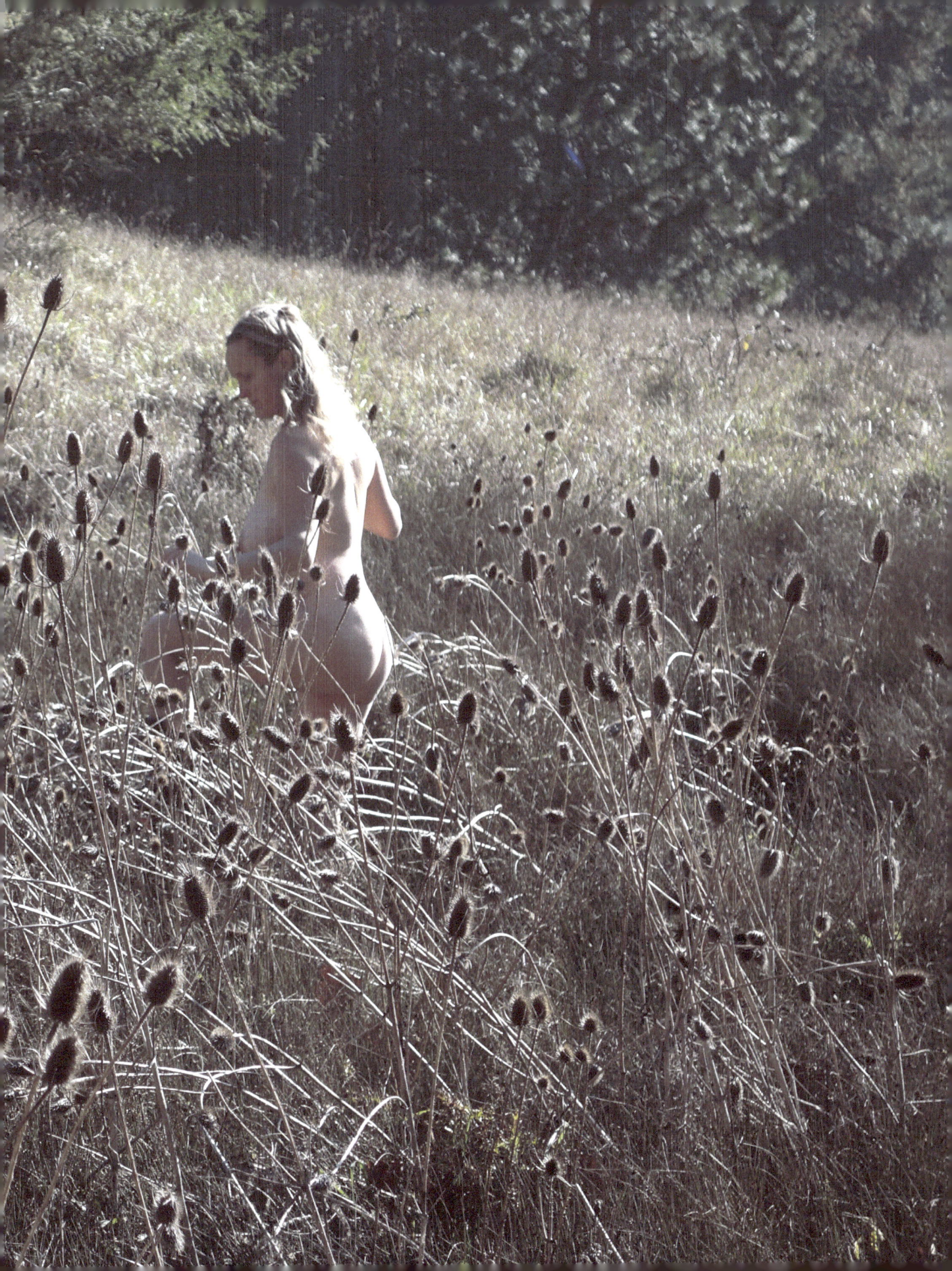

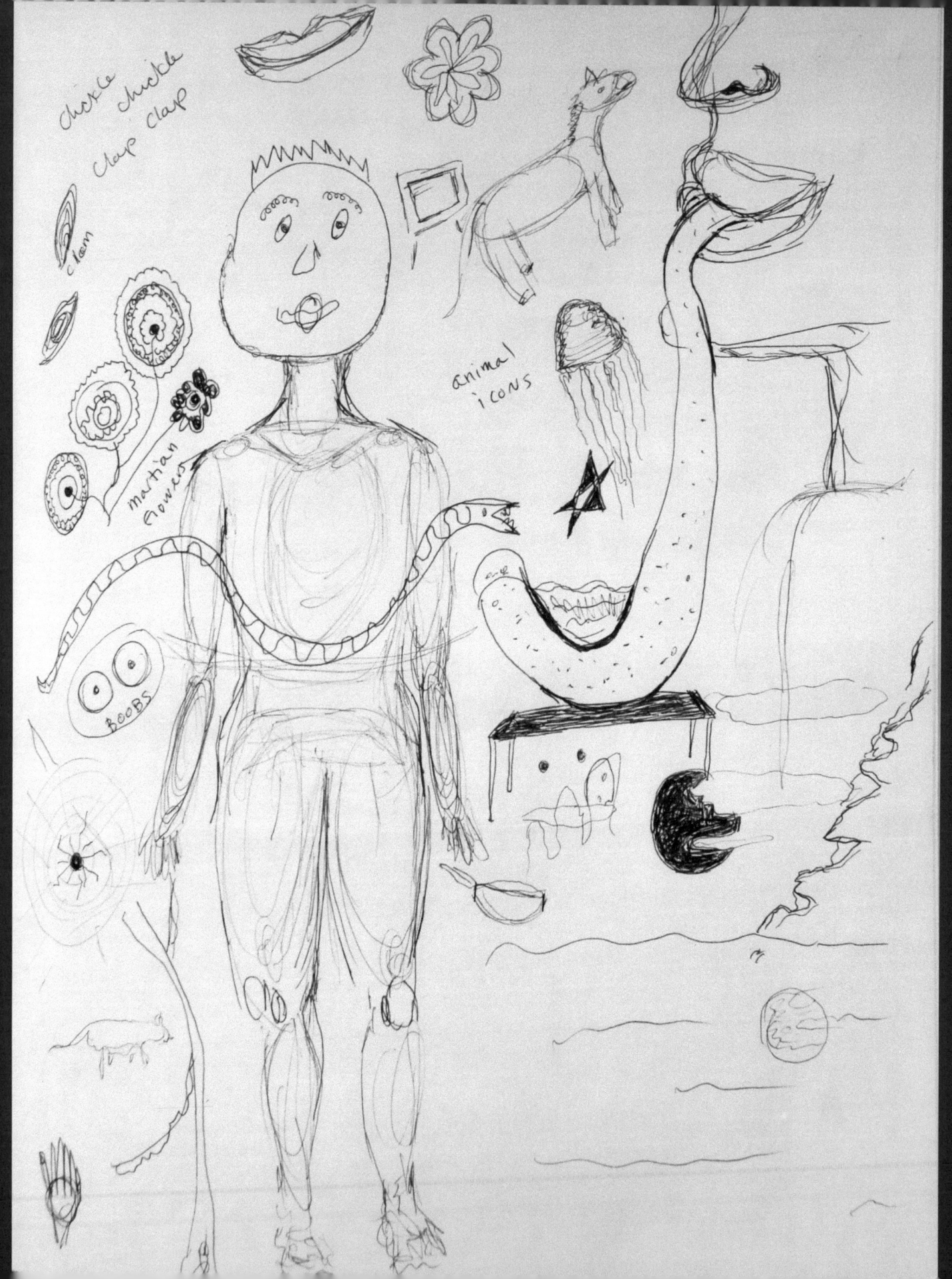

I keep thinking up all these different ideas +
one keep coming up repeatedly. The Sculpture.
idea ~ figurative stuff.

recycled
metals ~
woods

Symbols
WATER
FISH

Spirit lounger

ARE YOU
SCARED OF
YOUR ART?

Do you sometimes
JUST WANT TO BE
NORMAL?

ISOLATION FRIGHTENS YOU... Yet perhaps it is
important

SPECIAL IDEAS FOR Learning progressiy understandiy

SPACE

BODY ro

ROOTS
plants
sprouts
Flowers
FOOD
ocean
jovial   Fisy
Spirit octopus
Love   sand
        dirt
        soil
        waves
        wind
        air
        WATER
        FOOD
        Hair

crossin
into
unknow

SPIRIT
PICTURE

BLONDE
DADPY
LOVE

shiny
Bronze
balls

WOOD
+
metal

decompressed
chest

kittens
Dogs
animals

happy
spirits
with naNRA

New Beginnings

don't happen awake.

They happen **sleepless.**

A quick glimpse of

silver lakes and

flying magicians.

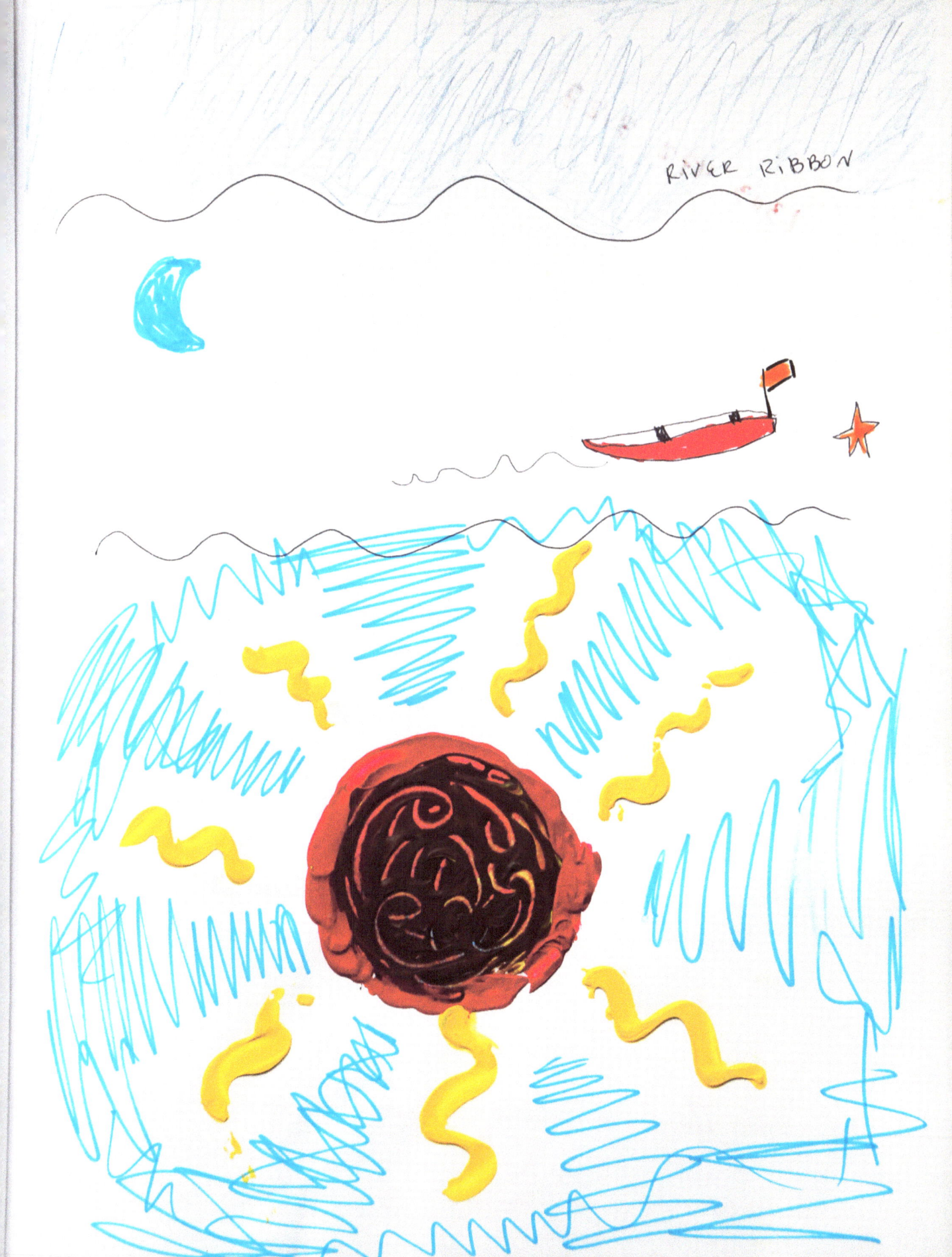

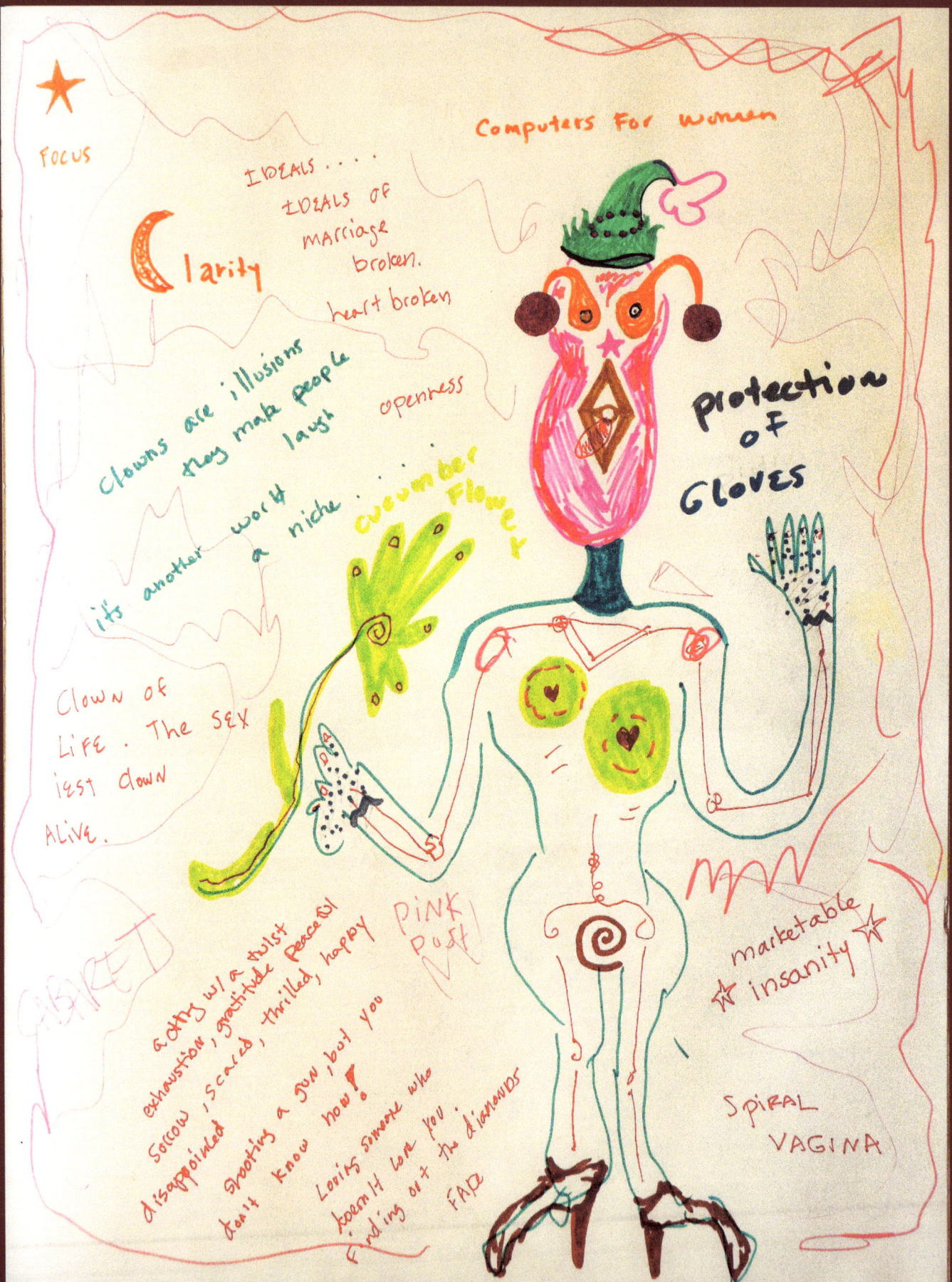

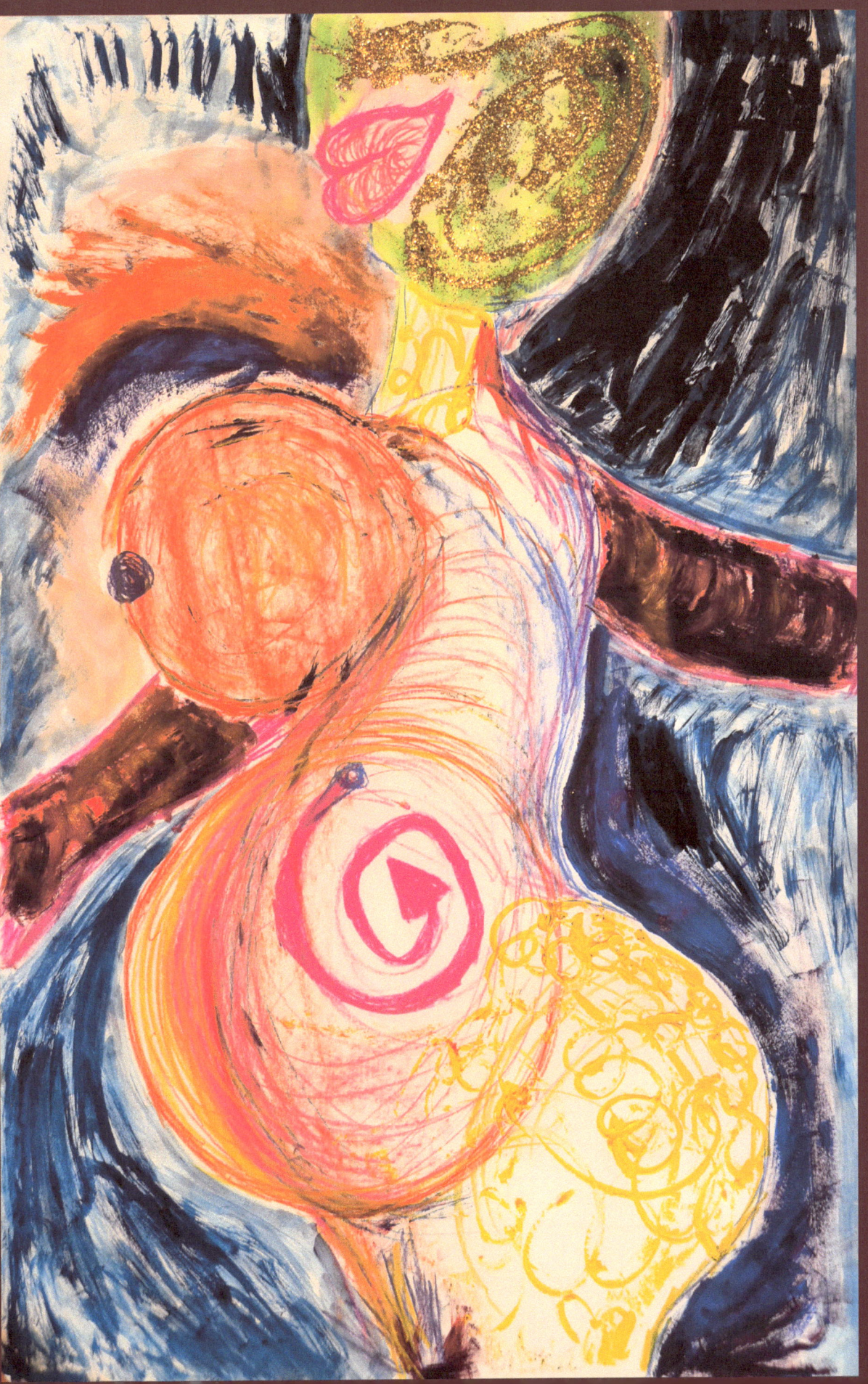

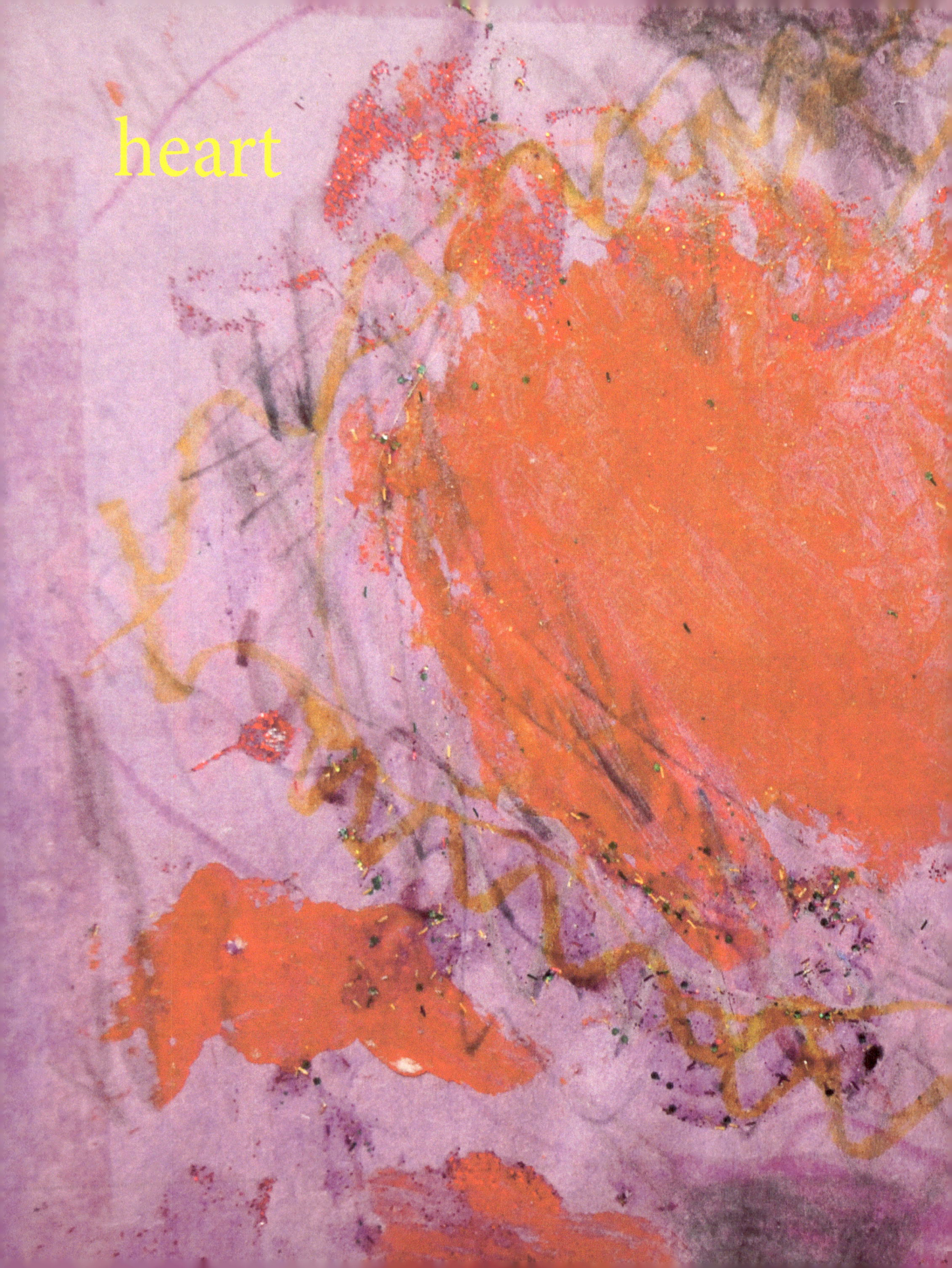

heart

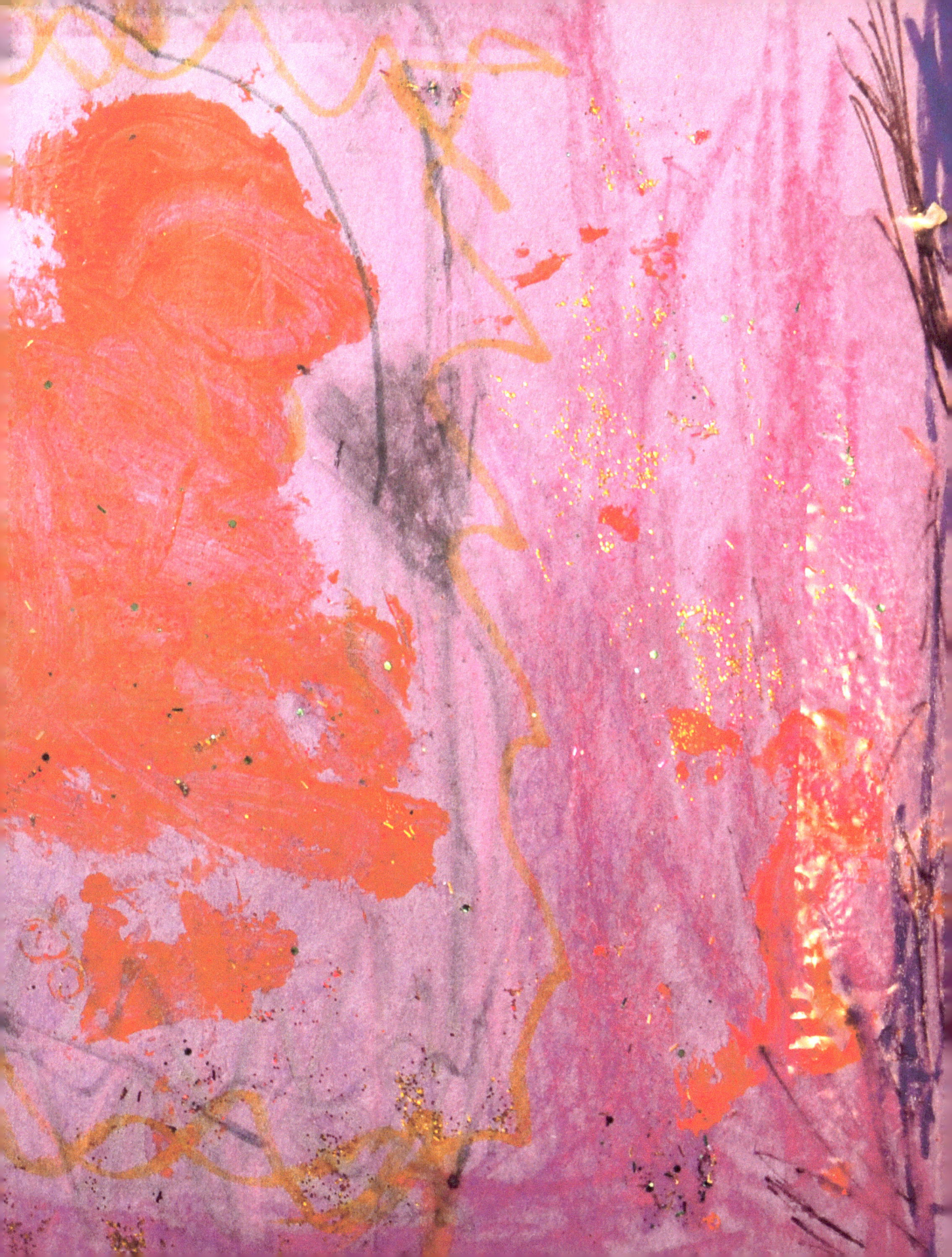

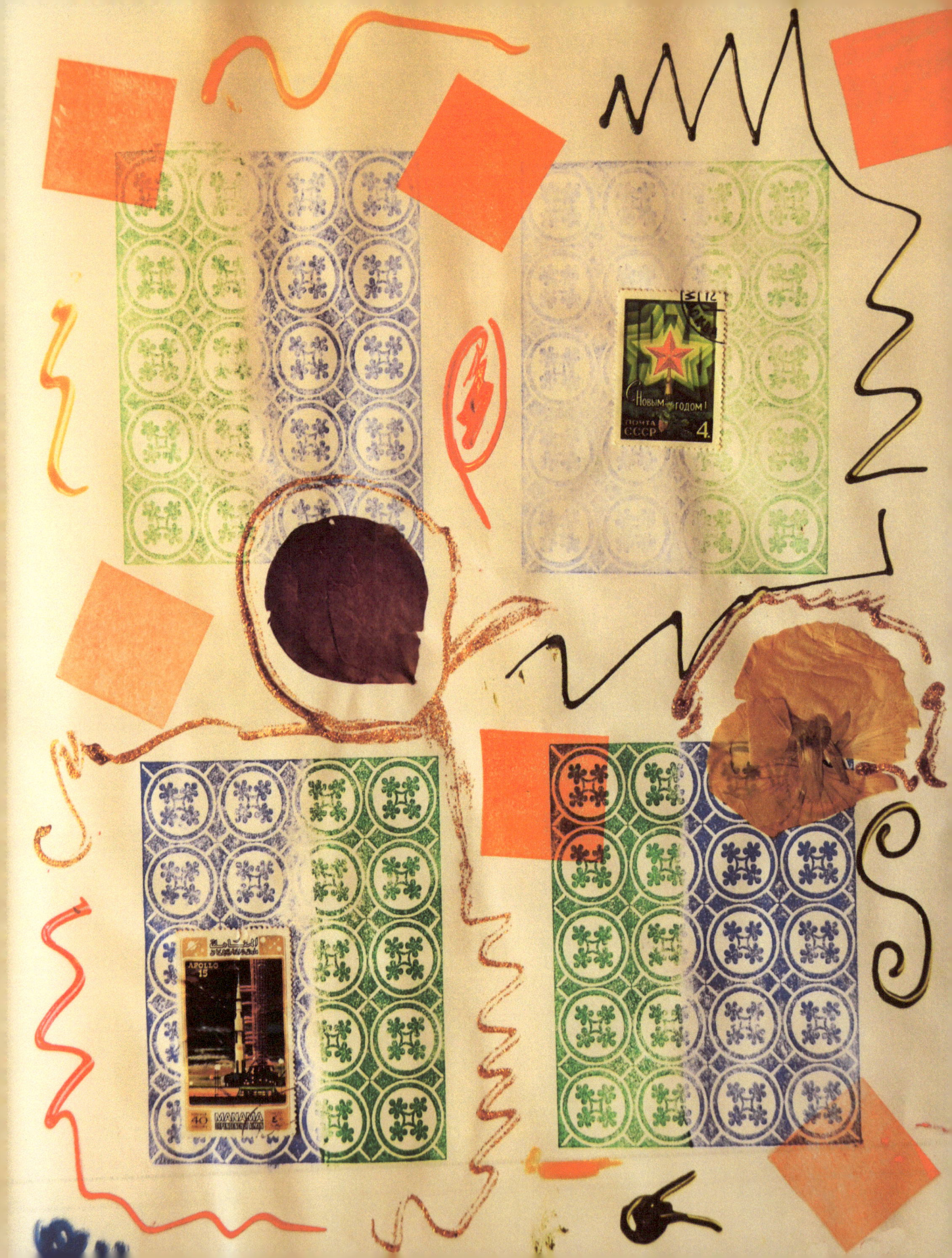

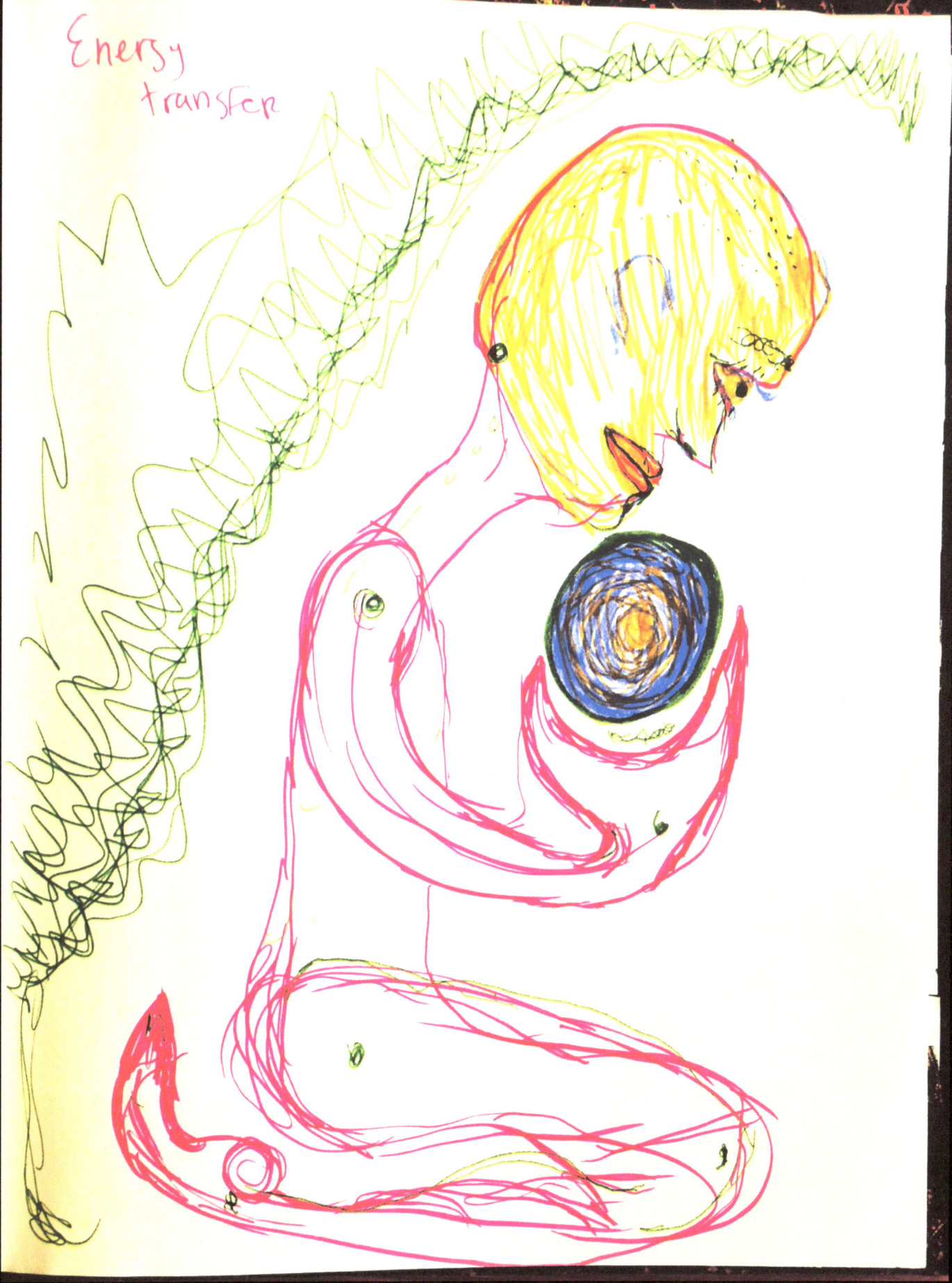

Sleep deprivation in creation is torture.

A baby comes, an idea in the middle of the night. A new relationship. BIRTH

Energy, pain, time.
My eyes are red, tattered.
Clipping, shuttering.

No longer wanting to be awake.
No choice.

I break down.
For the benefit of all.
I keep up with my duties.

having h
same wa
cleaned of
that was
wonder

, but she was a bimateria... ...spp
...at 18 which is why I gave it ain't just
after her. She sloppy. It was the work ethic
...hard for me ... no work ethic. I just
...ow that happens.

twang

tic

TONG

twit

TAZZLE

E

NOSE

cheek

• kisses •

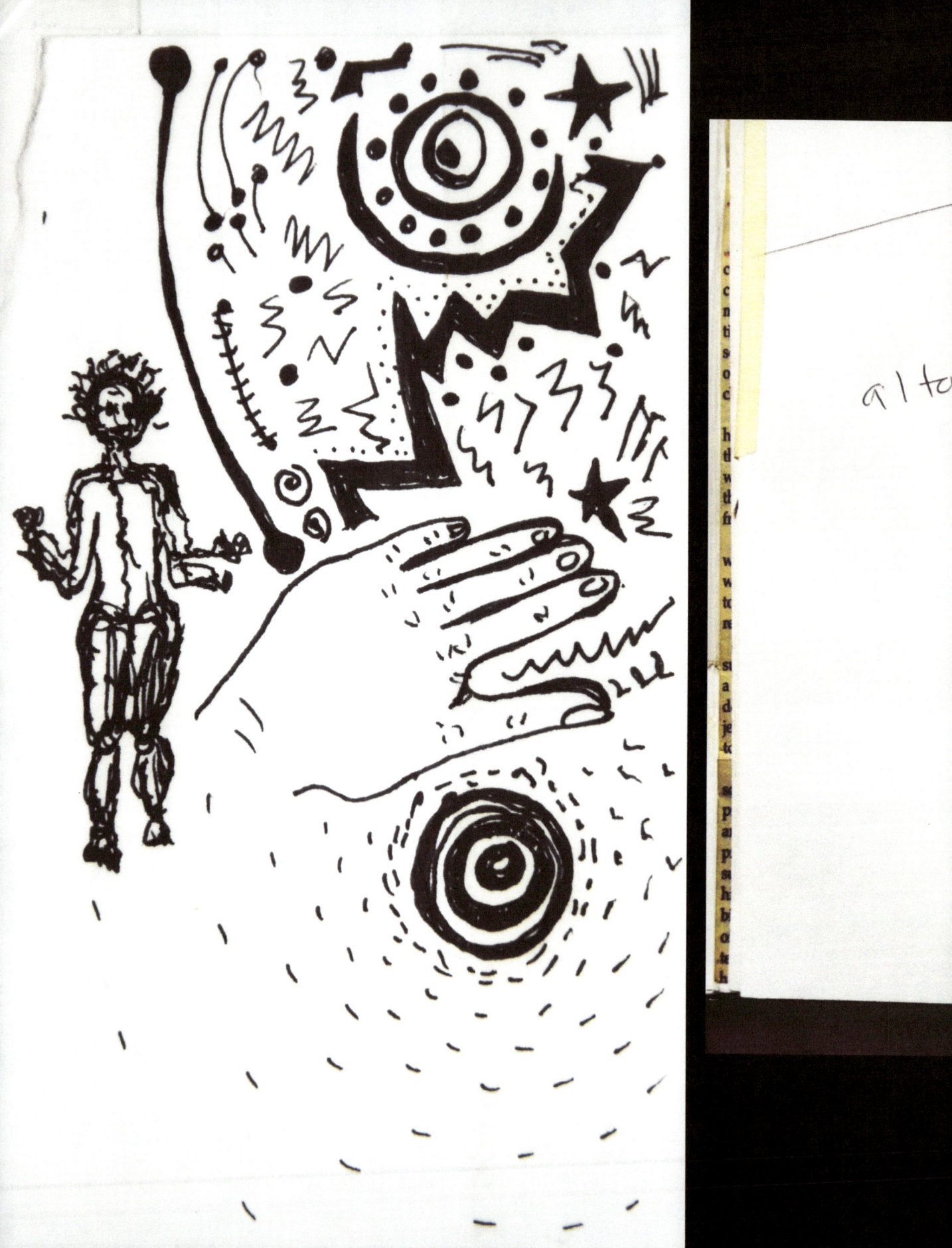

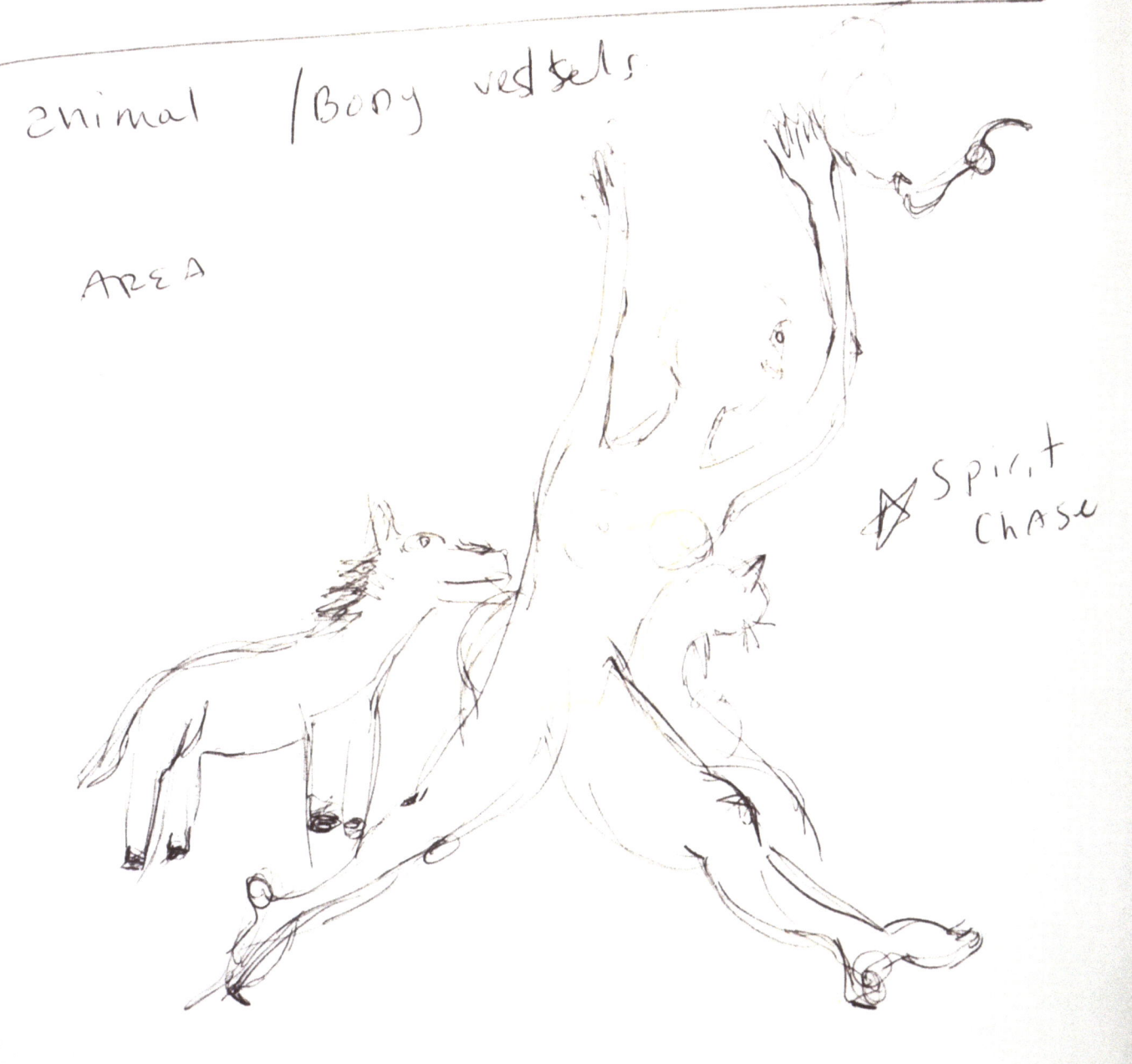

animal /Body vessels

AREA

Spirit Chase

Body Vessels

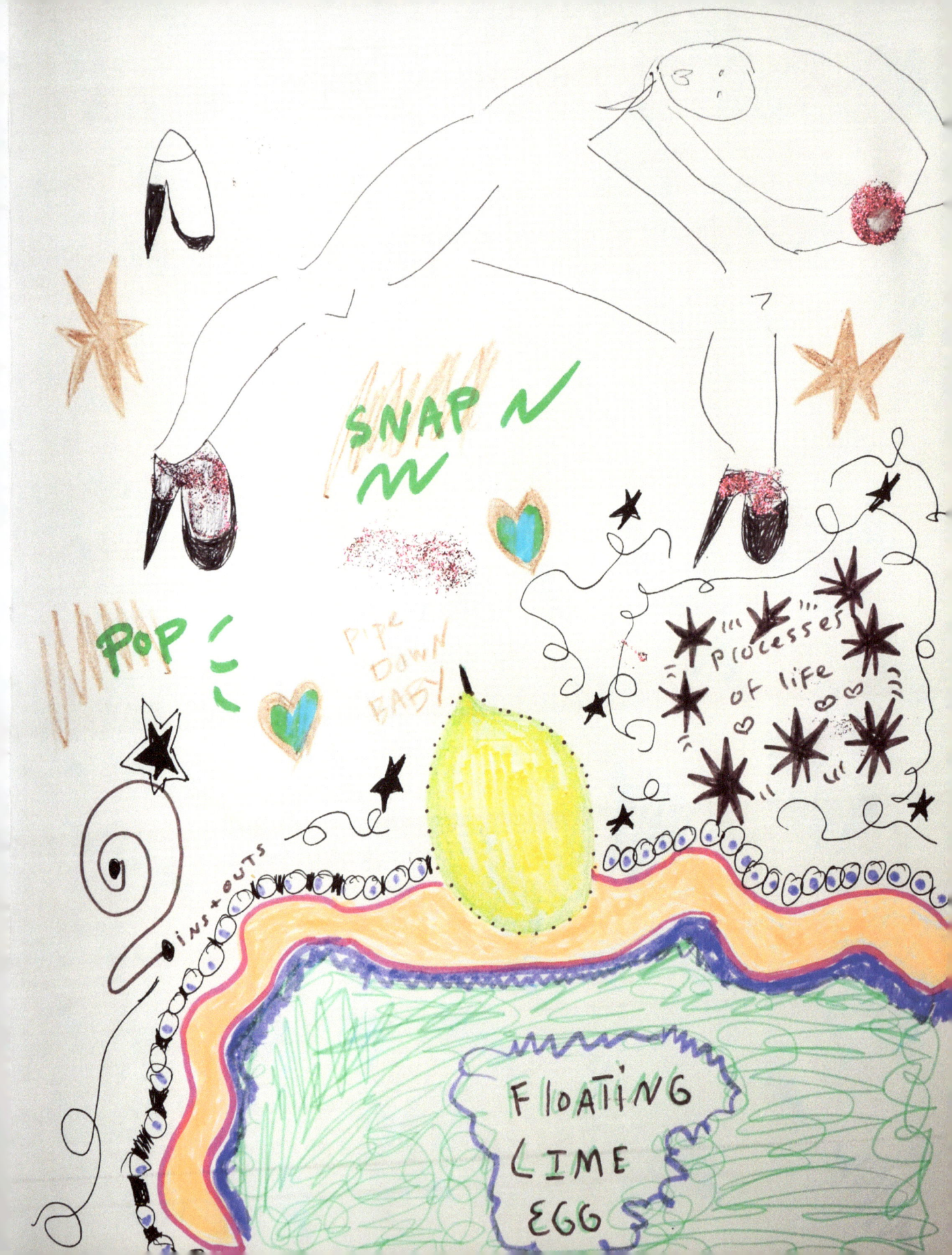

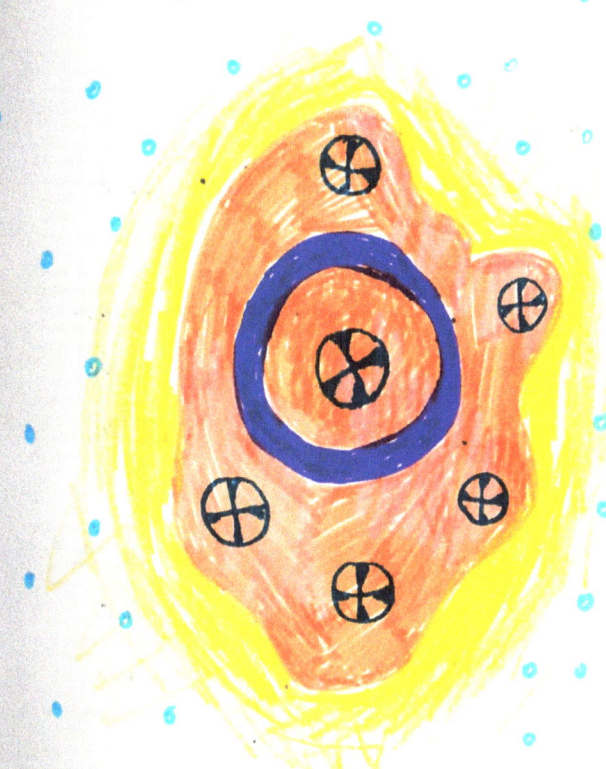

OUTER SPACE   EGG   MARCH 2012

Kept
in the
shadow
of a
former
self.
Where
to
turn
for help
and
re
assurance
??

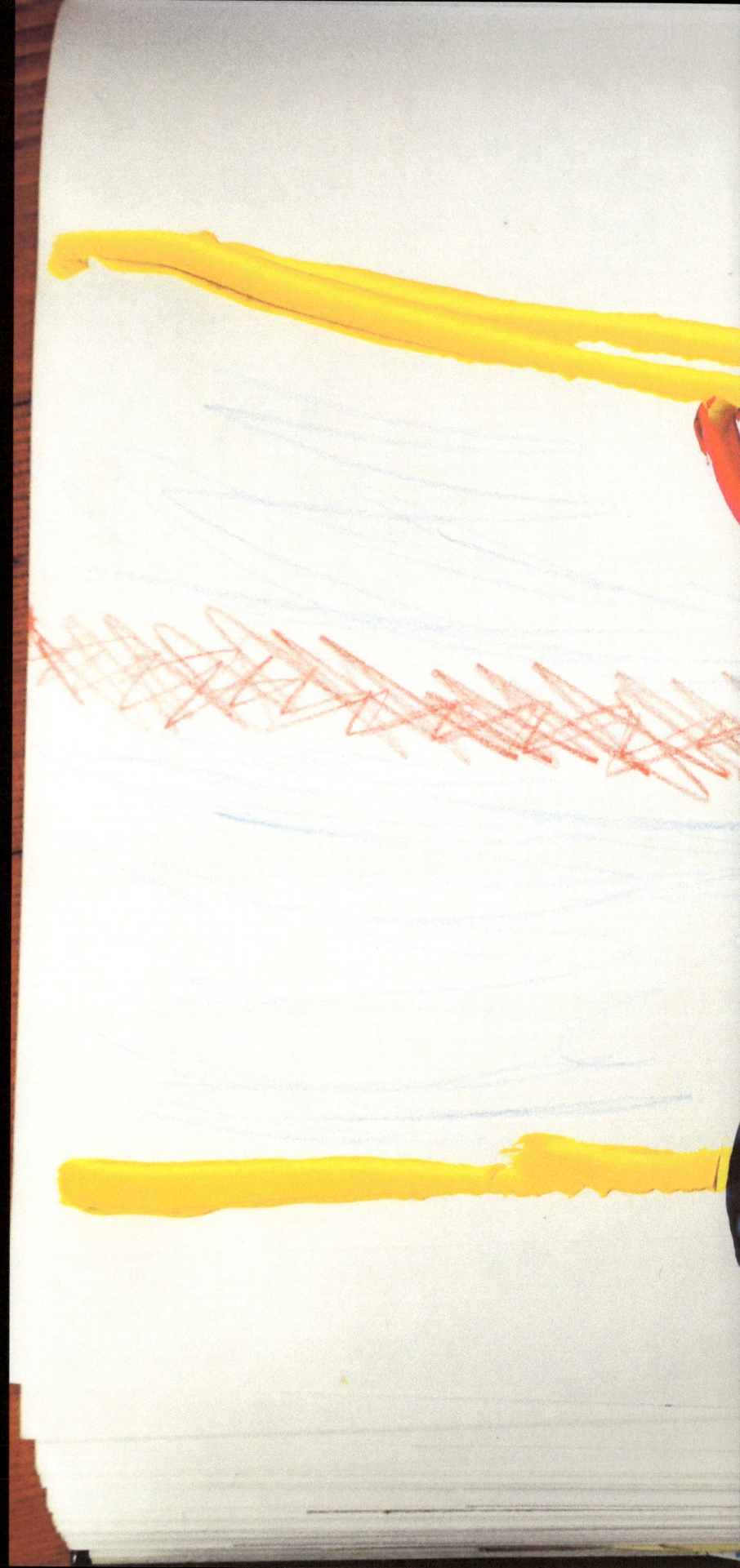

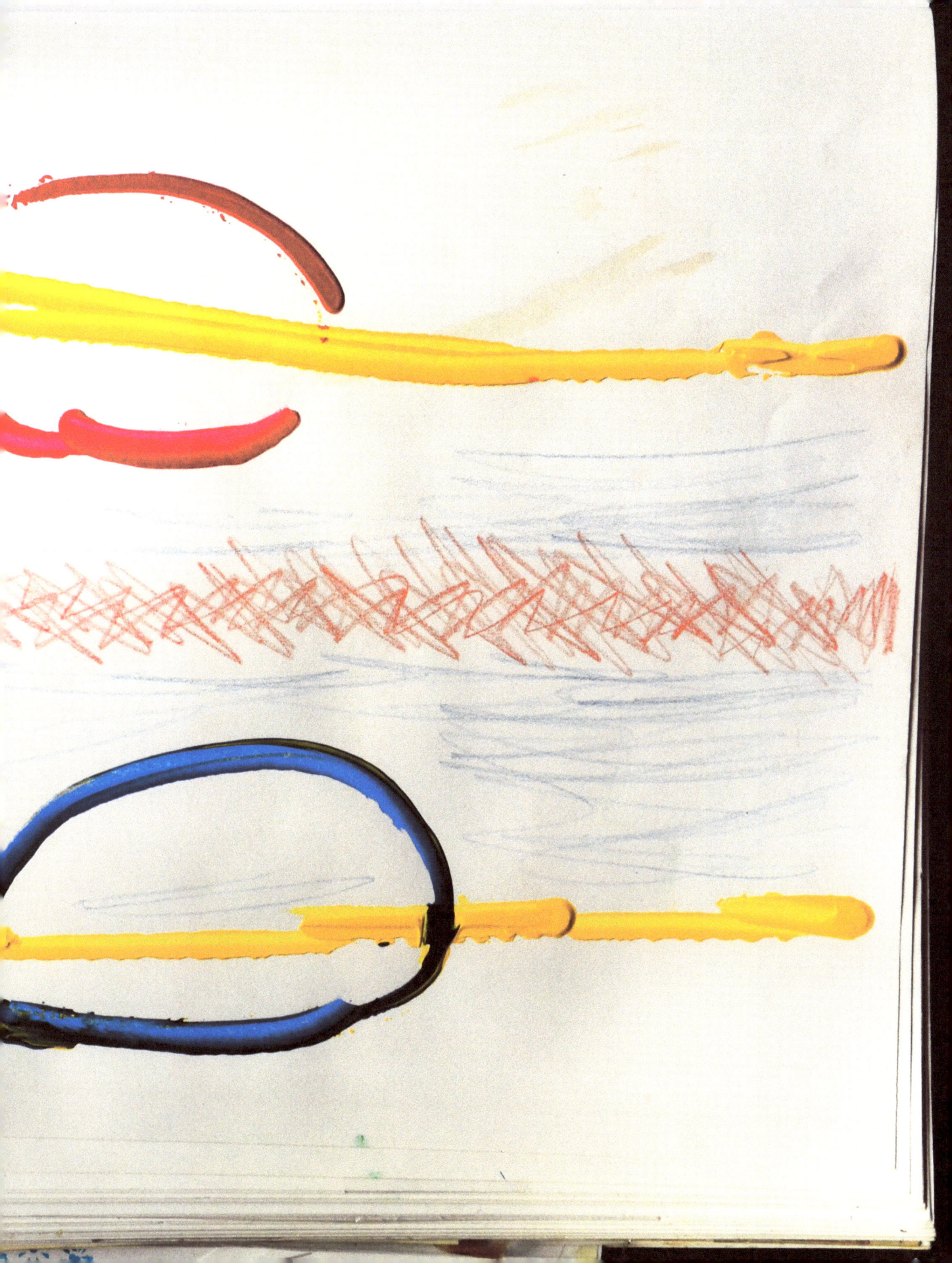

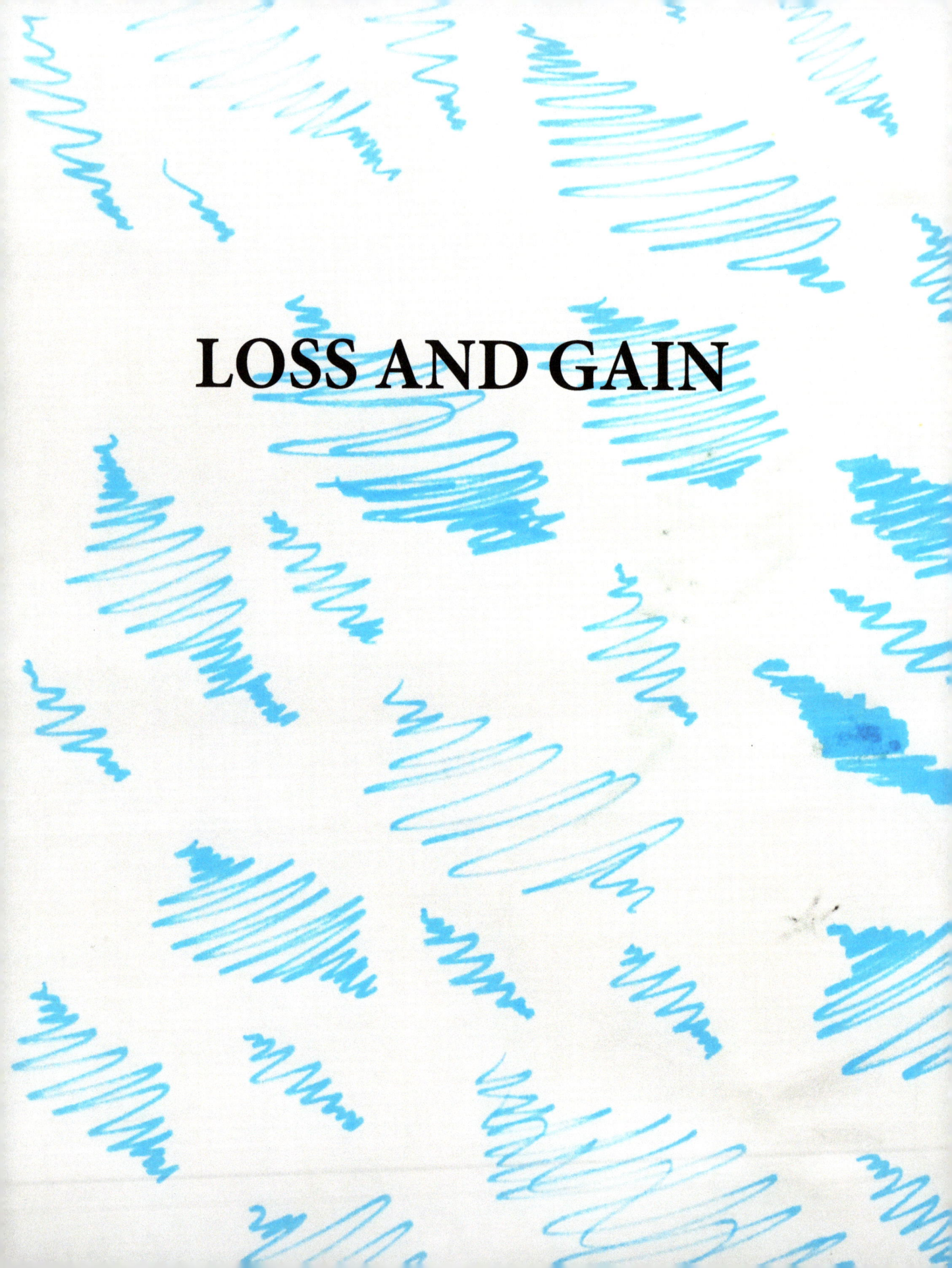

LOSS AND GAIN

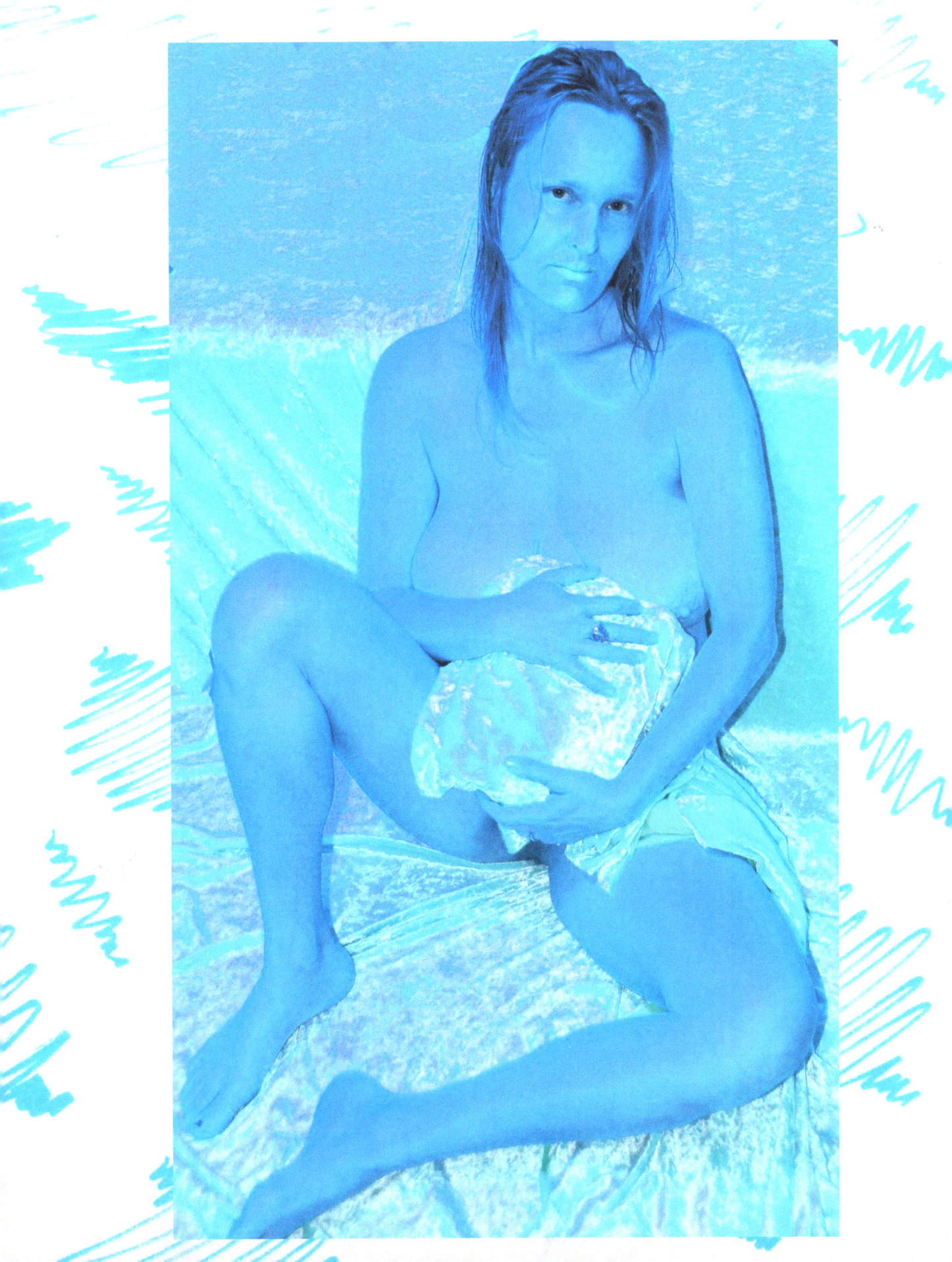

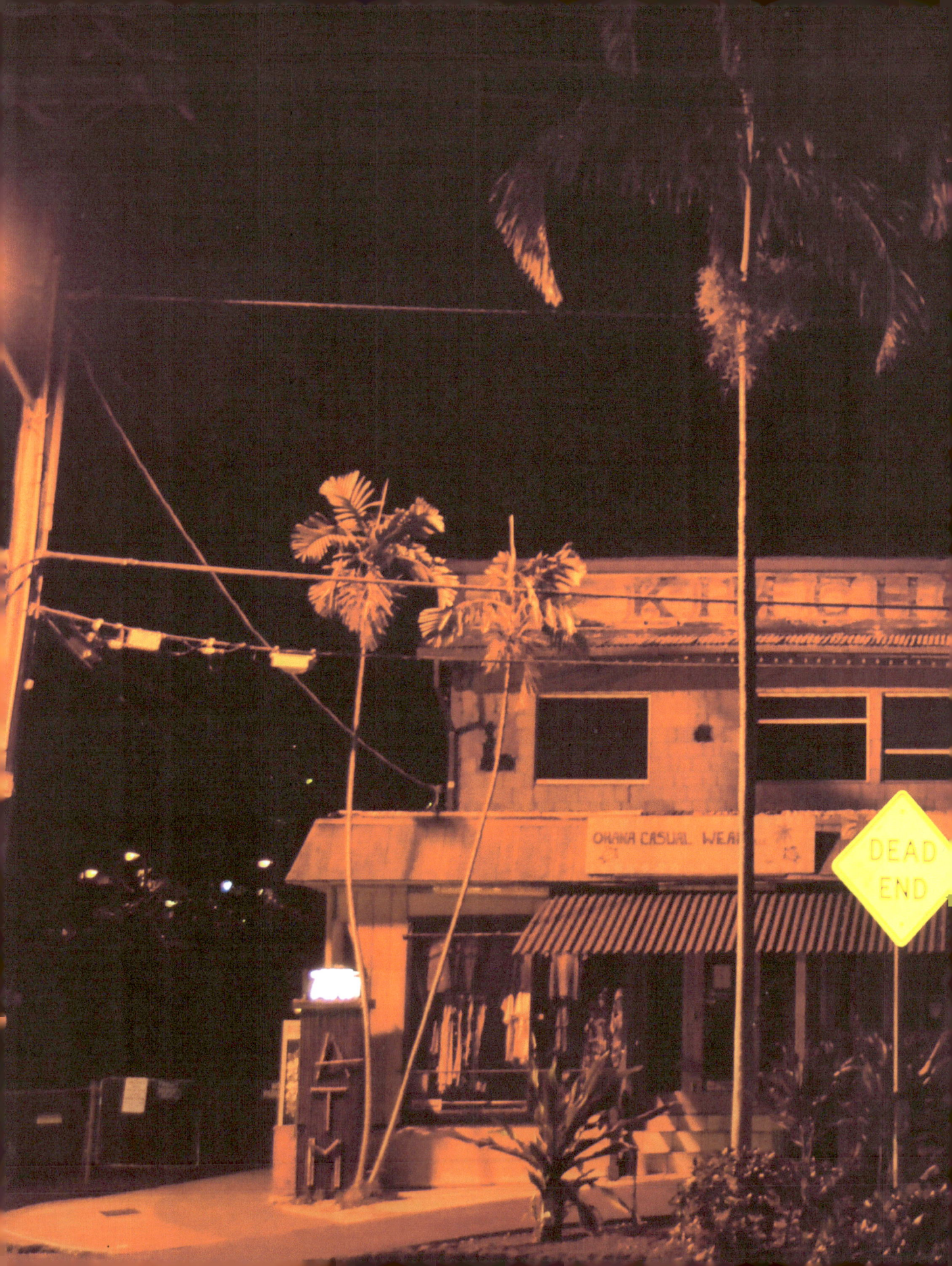

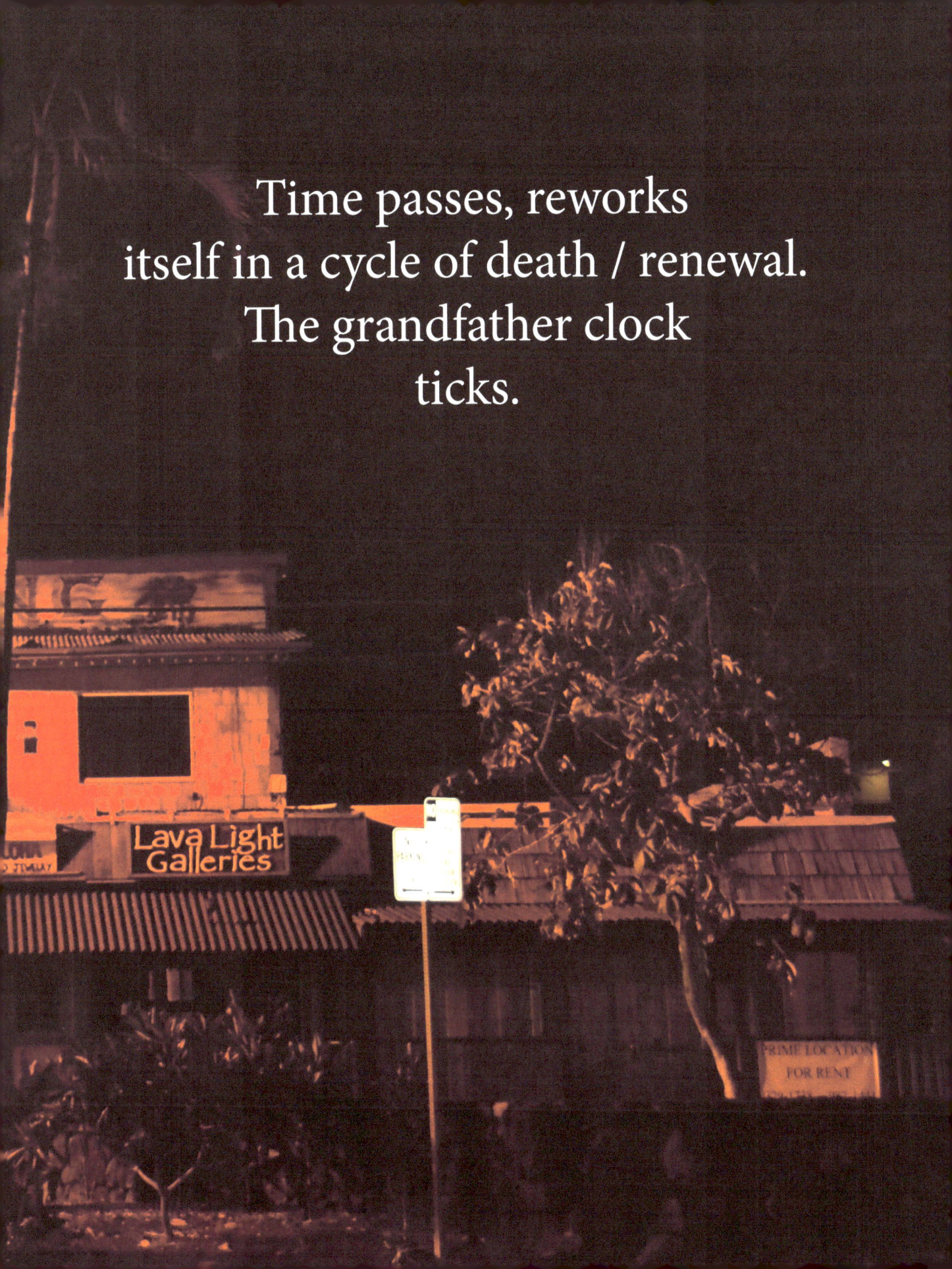

Time passes, reworks
itself in a cycle of death / renewal.
The grandfather clock
ticks.

Fighting a battle hidden
from the forefront.
Going out into the world
with new armory, a tattered
grin, and
green skin.
Sores, scars cover our inner
landscape. We trudge on.
Looking for
The Next Best Thing.

restraint

Armory

gusseted

Civil
soldier

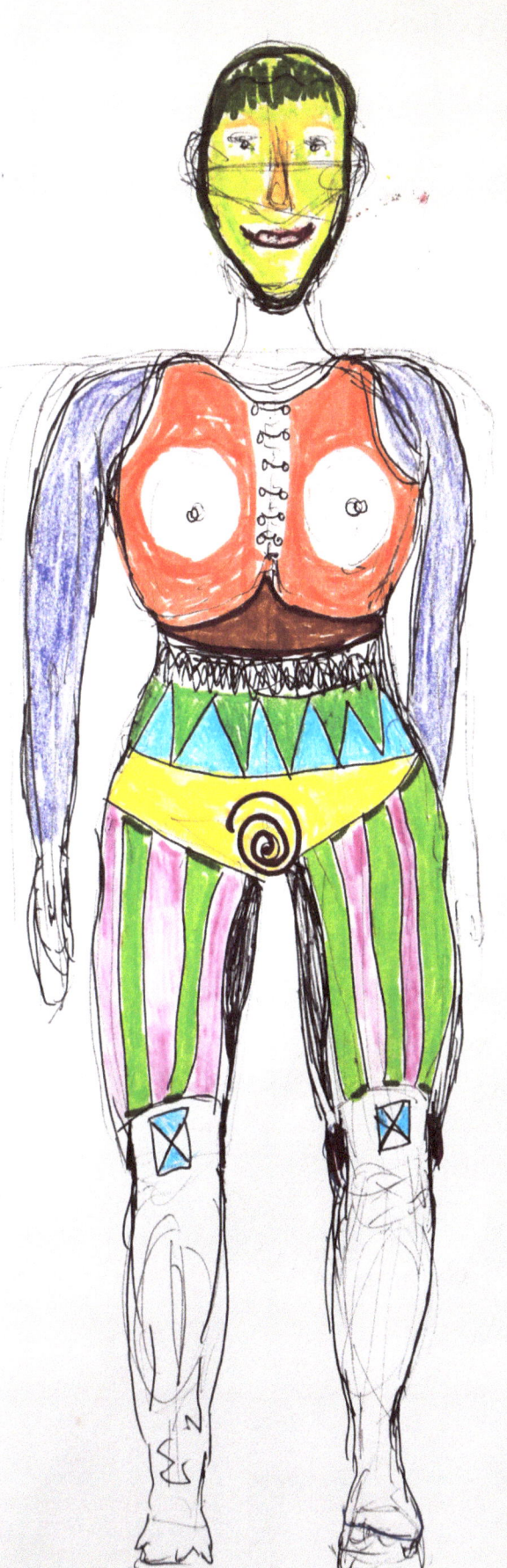

...lt around my daughter. I g

this wonderful life ... and

...off with her ... its neverer

want her t have more

city + people is Awesome. S

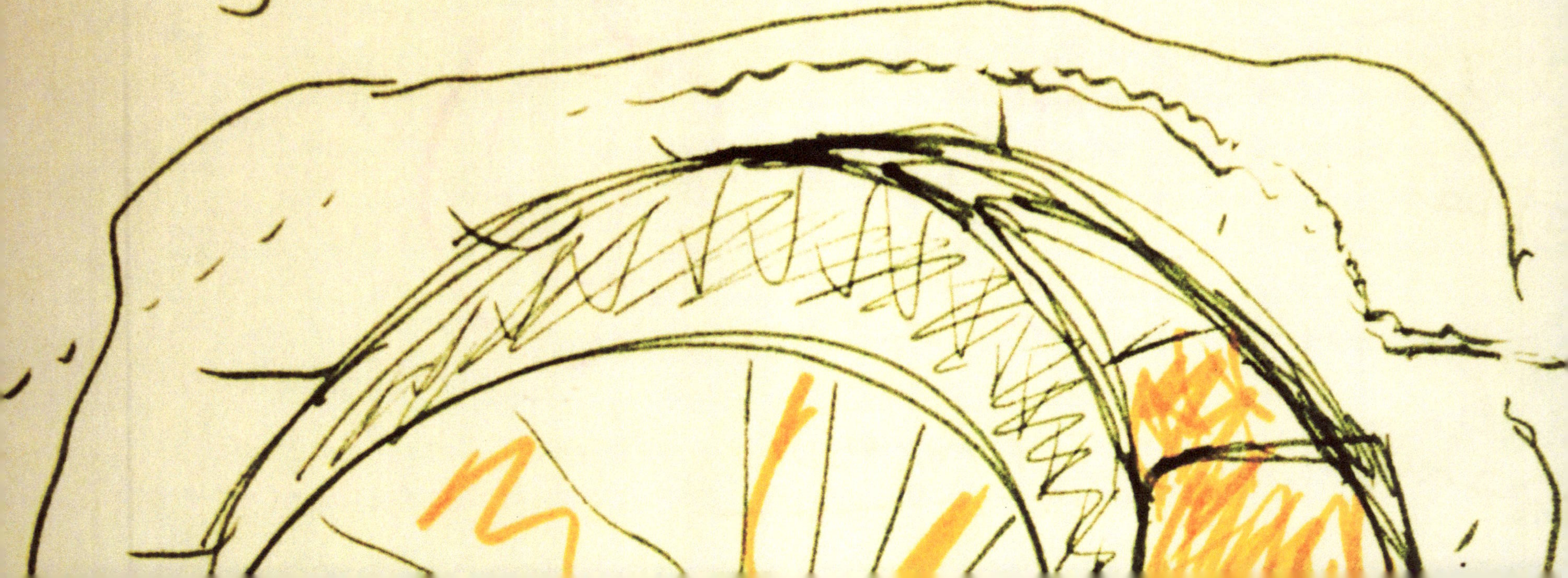

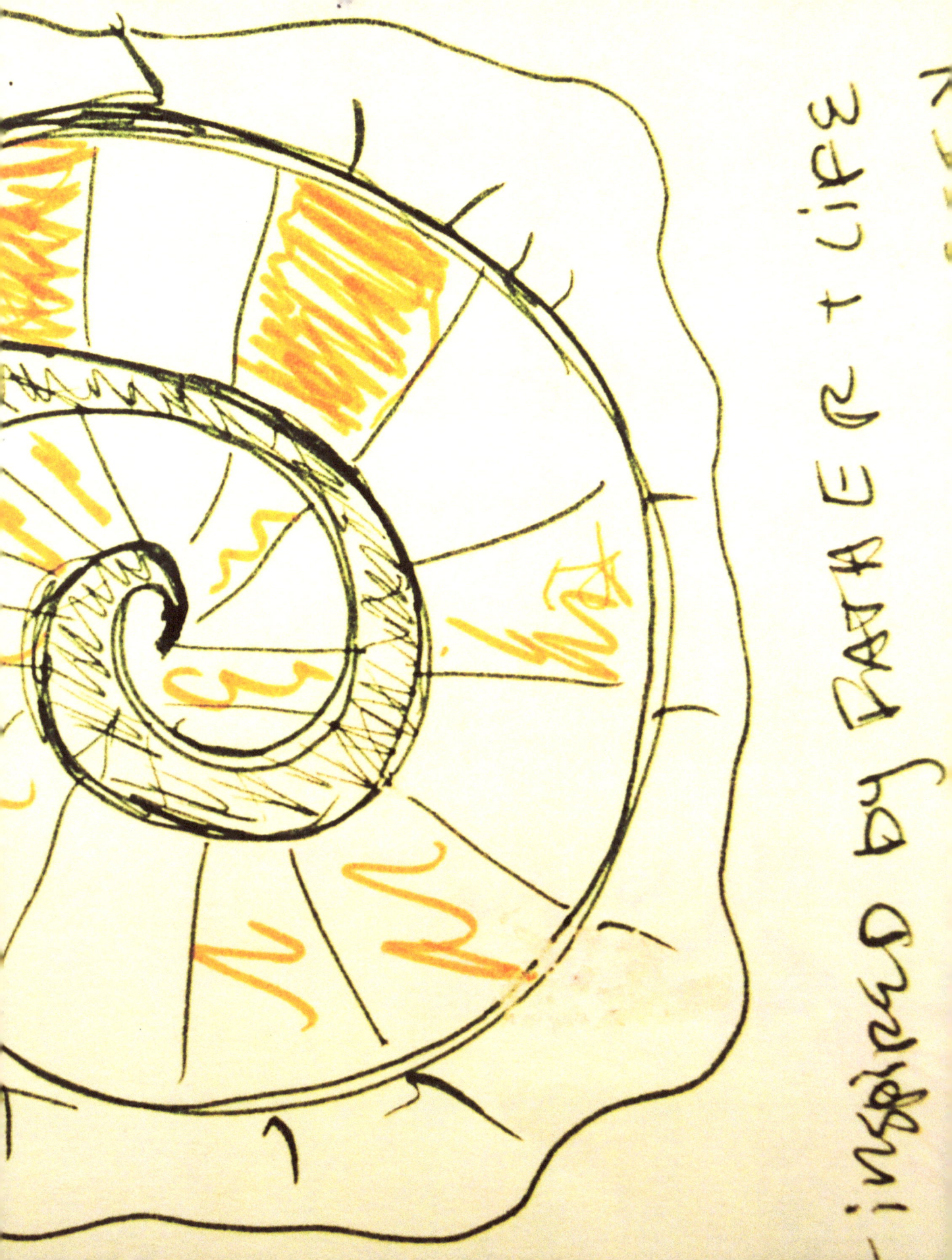

inspired by DAVID ERClift

Sophia Leah

deals with her
anguish and love through self-expression.
Born in
in Chicago, Illinois,
Sophia received a Bachelor of Science
degree in photography and sculpture
from Syracuse University
in New York.
Birth of The New is
art created
after giving birth to her first child.

Birth of The New
is her 4th published journal.

Sophia is now working on
her 5th published work:
WATER LOVE.

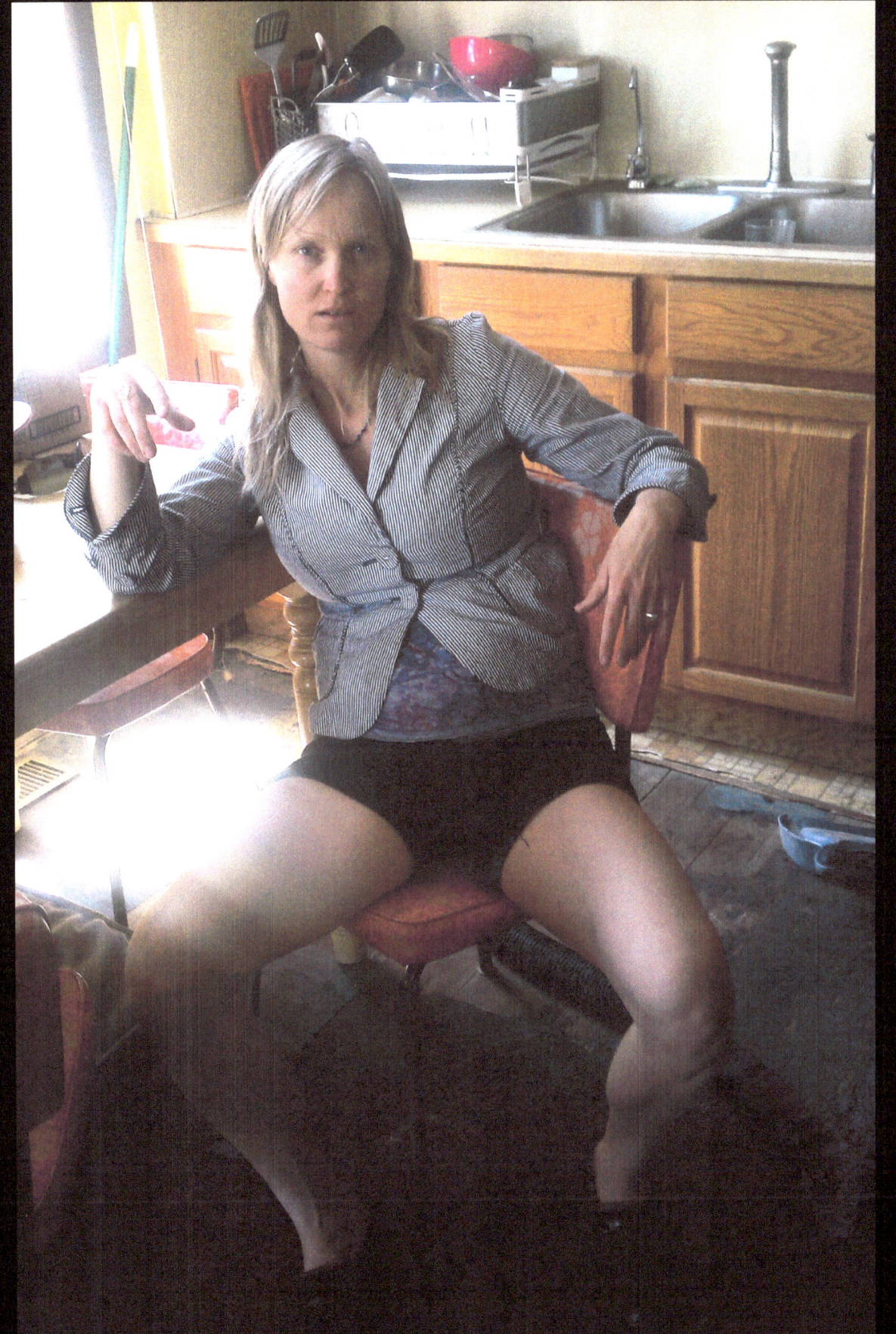